COOK THIS NOT THAT! SKINNY

COMFORT FOODS

BY DAVID ZINCZENKO AND MATT GOULDING

GALVAN!ZED Media

Printed in the United States.

Book design by George Karabotsos

Interior photo direction by Tara Long

Cover photos by Jeff Harris / Cover food styling by Ed Gabriels / Prop styling by Wendy Schelah
Photo producing by Ayla Christman

All interior photos by Thomas MacDonald and Mitch Mandel

Food styling by Diane Simone Vezza,
with the exception of pages 42–43, 174–175, 206–207, and 268–269, food styling by Melissa Reiss

Library of Congress Cataloging-in-Publication Data is on file with the publisher

ISBN-13: 978–1–940358-34-5   trade paperback

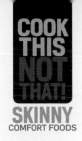

Dedication

To our moms, and moms everywhere,
who taught us everything we know about
the importance of a home-cooked meal.

—Dave and Matt

ACKNOWLEDGMENTS

We burned, scalded, singed, and sighed our way through hundreds of kitchen experiments (who knew comfort food could be so uncomfortable!) to bring you these recipes, but none of it would be possible without the incredible team we have supporting us every step of the way. In particular:

To George Karabotsos and his crew of crack designers, including Laura White, Elizabeth Neal, and Mark Michaelson. Above all, to Courtney Eltringham, who wrestled a jumble of recipes and sidebars into a beautiful book.

To Laura Pérez, who shopped, organized, sous cheffed, and taste-tested this book into being. You're the best. And to Clint Carter, Cathryne Keller, and Hannah McWilliams: This series would not be what it is without you. Thanks for everything you do.

To Tara Long: Your impeccable taste and unwavering vision continues to take these books to wonderful new places. And to her team, including Diane Vezza, Joan Parkin, Tom MacDonald, Nikki Weber, Mitch Mandel, Troy Schnyder, and Melissa Reiss: It's because of you that this food looks so good.

To our friends, families, and significant others: You've seen us sweat through quite a few of these, and still your support has never wavered. Maybe that's why we love cooking for you so much.

—Dave and Matt

Check out the other informative books in the **EAT THIS, NOT THAT!**®and **COOK THIS, NOT THAT!**™ series:

| Eat This, Not That! (2013) | Drink This, Not That! (2010) | Cook This, Not That! Kitchen Survival Guide (2010) | Grill This, Not That! Backyard Survival Guide (2012) | Eat This, Not That! Supermarket Survival Guide (2012) |

CONTENTS

Some folk are built like this, some folk are built like that

The way I'm built, now don't you call me fat

Because I'm built for comfort, I ain't built for speed

—Willie Dixon, "Built for Comfort"

Remember how simple and comforting food used
to be?

When you were a kid, there was nothing better than
waking up to a thick slice of French toast, maple syrup
and butter running over the edges, filling the kitchen
with the smell of autumnal goodness.

Or coming home from school to a thick wedge of
lasagna, the tangy sauce tickling your tongue and the
melted mozzarella stringing little spider webs between
your plate and fork.

Or taking a break from ice skating to linger over a
mug of hot chocolate, its little marshmallows floating on
top, keeping you warm on a cold winter's day.

Of course, that was then. You were a kid. You didn't
know any better. Now you're a grown-up, and when
you hear French toast, lasagna, and hot chocolate,
you think, Egads! Carbs! Saturated fats! Sugar! I can't
eat that!

Being a grown-up sucks, doesn't it?

Well, this book is about to change all that. *Eat This,
Not That! Skinny Comfort Foods* is like a high school
reunion where only the kids you really liked show up.
Steamed Broccoli? Couldn't make it.

Tofu? Not invited. Lima Beans? Serving a 6-month prison term for DWIF—Dining Without Intoxicating Flavor. You won't find any of those bullies and bums in here.

But Fettuccine with Turkey Bolognese, Molten Chocolate Cake, and those old jokers, Mac and Cheese? They're all waiting for you inside. My goal is to get you reacquainted with your very best friends from childhood—some close buddies that maybe you grew a little wary of over the years, but you never stopped missing, never stopped thinking about.

Sounds great, you're thinking. But I'm a grown-up now, and I have grown-up concerns, like the refined carbs and the trans fats and the sugars and the glycemic index and . . . ahhhhh!

Well, yes, we are grown-ups now, and watching our weight is more important than ever before. That's why *Skinny Comfort Foods* is here, to make all your favorites a lot less scary—and to help you lose weight, eat great, and start enjoying the company of some wonderful old friends.

Stop Stressing, Start Indulging

In reality, a lot of the foods we remember from childhood weren't necessarily all that bad for us—at least, back when we were kids. What's happened is that food processors and chain restaurants decided that the foods we already loved needed to be "improved," and so starting in the '70s and increasingly through the '80s, they started "improving" them by adding new kinds of sugars and other chemicals, turning misdemeanor indulgences into nutritional felonies.

CONSIDER THIS: How much high fructose corn syrup did you eat today?

Your answer: Uh, none?

CORRECT ANSWER: If you're an average American, you ate 12 teaspoons' worth. That would be just today. It was probably in the sauce you tossed with your spaghetti, the ketchup you spread on your burger (and the bun as well), the bread your turkey sandwich came on, and the iced tea you washed it down with.

But you don't need to be downing a chemical cocktail of bad-for-you stuff every time you crave the comfort of your old food friends. And you don't have to live on a diet of romaine lettuce and kidney beans to start dropping pounds and keep them off forever. In fact, you can run for comfort any time you want—and still lose 10, 20, 30 pounds or more. All you need are a few smart swaps, and a quiver of simple recipes. Once you know a handful of secrets, you'll be indulging in all your favorite comfort foods, and watching the pounds disappear.

Before we get started, however, it's worth answering one question: What exactly is "comfort food"?

The first thing you might think of is that creamy tomato soup Grandma made for you when you came in with a chill from building a snowman in the backyard; the mac and cheese Mom cooked up when you got the mumps in fourth grade; the chocolate brownie sundaes that you and your friends shared after you got dumped by that loser they all warned you about. Comfort food is about memories, right?

In part, yes. The taste of melting American cheese on your tongue, the smell of apple pie cooling on the counter, the sound of Mom clanking the pots and pans in the kitchen while Dad sits in the living room, cursing the Red Sox—they trigger our memories, and when we recall happier, more innocent times, we can't help but feel more at peace. It's the reason you can still hear The Oldies from the '50s and even earlier on radio stations every Sunday.

But there's actually a science to comfort food, and to why we crave what we crave when we're stressed or blue, that has

nothing to do with Mom's cooking or Dad's scatological references to Fenway Park. Let me tell you what happens, in part, when we eat comfort foods, and the biological reason why your college roommate's tofu and lentil stew never quite satisfied those emotional needs.

The Science of Comfort Food

I don't know about you, but I could pretty much use some comforting all the time. If it's sweet, fatty, greasy, chewy, or just plain yummy, I'm ready to run into its arms.

That's because, like you and everyone else living in the USA right now, I'm chronically stressed. I probably manage about 500 emails a day, several dozen phone calls, and a few dozen texts. Then there are the Tweets, the friend requests, and the myriad other social media coming at me with the intensity of a 4-year-old on a Butterfinger binge—and that's before I even walk to my mailbox.

That stress triggers the release of several hormones, starting with two main ones, adrenaline and cortisol. Adrenaline you know—it's the stuff that gets your heart racing and your blood pumping and your wallet opening for yet another superhero movie. Nothing wrong with that: The occasional adrenaline rush is what makes life worth living, after all.

But the other hormone, cortisol, is the real problem. What it's supposed to do is release fat and sugar into your bloodstream, so you can run away from the snarling sabertooth or the attacking alligator or the uncaged Kardashian or whatever other primitive man-eating predator is on your tail. But when stress becomes chronic— when the untamed tiger is replaced by a daily onslaught of rising bills, mindless tasks, and disheartening remarks from the boss—cortisol can actually signal your cells to store as much fat as possible and inhibit the body from releasing fat to burn as energy. What's worse, that fat tends to accumulate in the abdominal region, because visceral fat, which resides behind the abdominal muscles, has more cortisol receptors than fat below the skin.

I know what you're thinking: What does this have to do with Grandma's creamy tomato soup?

Well, our hormonal reactions to stress

4 REASONS TO SPEND MORE TIME IN THE

CUTTING CALORIES HAS A BIGGER IMPACT THAN BURNING CALORIES

In a meta-analysis of 33 clinical trials, Brazilian scientists determined that diet controls about 75 percent of weight loss. Working out helps, of course, but a smart eating plan will get you three-fourths of the way there without your ever having to break a sweat. (That's the difference between six-pack and eight-pack abs!) Another study published by the Public Library of Science found that women who worked out with a trainer for 6 months lost no more weight than those who merely filled out health forms—in other words, those who started thinking about what they were eating. You can do that easily. As soon as you start cooking, you become instantly aware of everything on your plate.

FORCING YOURSELF INTO THE GYM INCREASES YOUR LIKELIHOOD OF INDULGING LATER

Some researchers have compared will-power to muscle—once you work it hard, it becomes weak. So by forcing yourself into the gym today—when you don't really have the time—you're setting yourself up to fail tomorrow when you're confronted with milk shakes, french fries, and chimichan-gas. Unfortunately, it takes only one slip to negate an entire sweat session. Ever reward a trip to the gym with some food outside your normal eating regime? Sure, we all have. But the truth is, we're probably better off sticking to home-cooked food and skipping the gym.

help explain why we develop cravings for fried chicken, chocolate chip cookies, grilled cheese, chicken soup, apple pie, and the like whenever we're feeling like we need a hug.

To qualify as comfort food, a meal needs to be easy to eat, and it needs to be high in fat. In a study published in the *Journal of Clinical Investigation,* University of Texas researchers exposed mice to a chronically high level of stress and discovered that their bodies manufactured an increased amount of the hunger hormone ghrelin. Not only that, but the frantic furry subjects

also showed a corresponding increase in their preference for—and intake of—high-fat food.

So we not only crave comfort food when we're sad, we are actually hormonally triggered to eat more of it! That's one reason why, in a British study in the journal *Obesity,* adolescents who reported greater levels of stress had higher BMIs and greater waist circumferences compared to teens with less perceived stress.

And obesity and stress are a lethal one-two punch. You already know that carrying

KITCHEN THAN YOU DO IN THE GYM

IT TAKES LESS TIME TO COOK IN THAN IT DOES TO WORK OUT

You can eat a 1,000-calorie fast-food burger in 5 minutes, but you'll spend an hour or more burning it off at the gym. And that's if you're busting your butt. Now imagine that you decided instead to skip the burger and forgo the gym. You could head home and, in about 20 minutes, you could have a juicier, tastier, 350-calorie cheeseburger made with the finest ingredients and seasoned just the way you like it. Will the portion be smaller? Probably, but so what? Cornell University research shows that eating satisfaction is derived from the flavor intensity and visual impact of a meal, not necessarily the amount served. Plus, you're left with extra cash in your wallet, you've saved 45 minutes, and you've "burned" more than 600 calories.

YOU CAN WORK EXERCISE INTO YOUR DAILY ROUTINE

Think of all the opportunities you have to be active throughout the day. Do you take advantage? Try taking the stairs over the elevator, walking across the office instead of sending an e-mail, or riding a bike instead of taking a cab. In essence, you can cheat your gym session. But food? There's no cheating there; it's only good when it's made fresh. Researchers at the University of Minnesota determined that compared with cooking for yourself, consuming more restaurant and ready-made meals—think frozen dinners and carryout—could have a negative impact on your overall health. So food should come first, and dedicated gym time second.

too many pounds can put you at risk for every disease under the sun. But check this out: In a study at the University of Western Ontario, researchers took hair follicles from 100 men, half of whom were recently hospitalized for heart attacks. (Which is exactly what you want to have happen to you after you've just had a heart attack.) The upshot: The men who'd suffered a cardiac episode had higher cortisol levels in their hair—a direct link between stress and The Big One.

So the plan is obvious: Turn off the phone, shut down the computer, move into a cave, and never eat a slice of meat loaf again. Right?

Well, that's one answer. But we think we have a better one.

Take Comfort— and Lose Weight!

We all deserve the right to make ourselves feel better. And the crazy thing is, chasing our blues with comfort foods is scientifically proven to work, at least in the short term.

In a somewhat bizarre study in 2011, participants had their stomachs filled with either saline solution or saturated fat. Then they were shown images of sad faces and made to listen to sad music. (Apparently, the researchers had a vast collection of Dan Fogelberg records.) Compared to the moods of those who had only salt water in their guts, the subjects who had a belly full of fat reported feeling less miserable. When we're faced with negative circumstances, fatty foods literally comfort us.

But constantly filling your belly with fat—especially when stress-related cortisol is triggering your body to store more of that fat around your middle—isn't exactly a great long-term strategy for feeling better. And when stress enters our lives, it not only plays havoc with our diets and our health, but it impacts the eating habits of those around us as well. In another study in the journal *Social Science & Medicine*, parents who had higher work-life stress levels were more likely to come home to a less healthful family food environment and a higher family intake of sugar-sweetened beverages and fast-food items.

So comfort foods are the ultimate catch-22: They help us manage stress and sadness, while they make us fat and unhealthy, causing us more stress and sadness.

But there's an answer, and it's in these pages: Skinny Comfort Food. If you could capture the rich, creamy goodness of your favorite feel-good foods, keep all the delicious flavor and that chewy, gooey mouthfeel, and yet dramatically reduce the calories, then you'd be able to indulge your cravings whenever you felt the desire.

And that's our goal. My coauthor, *New York Times* best-selling food journalist and trained chef Matt Goulding, and I have dissected some of the most popular comfort foods on the market. And what we discovered is that many of them are loaded with extra fat and calories that aren't at all necessary for tickling our taste buds or triggering those feel-good hormones.

For example:

> Let's say a bad day at work has you craving a juicy cheeseburger. You could stop in at sit-down restaurant for an avocado turkey burger (it's turkey, how bad could it be?). But you'd be drowning your sorrows in 54 grams of fat, amongst the 908 calories you'd down—before you even ate the first french fry. But try our Southwest Turkey Burger recipe on page 136 and save 438 calories and 28 grams of fat!

> Another stressful day with the kids turns a young parent's mind to . . . chocolate cake. A typical restaurant cake will cost you 1,110 calories and 59 grams of fat. Turn to page 344, however, and you'll discover how to enjoy the same gooey, chocolaty awesomeness for just 320 calories.

> What's a scary movie marathon without pizza to snack on? (Food that can't be spilled is always the best choice for Wes Craven fans.) But order in a Pizza Hut Italian Sausage Pan Pizza, and it won't be just the actors on the TV who are walking around like zombies. Just two slices will deliver 780 calories. Check out our recipe on page 158, and learn how to make a pie that cuts those calories nearly in half.

What's the upshot? You'll have just saved yourself 1,548 calories by eating pizza, a cheeseburger, and chocolate cake. Just making those simple swaps twice a week could strip away 45 pounds in the next year!

So what do you say? Are you ready to start taking comfort in food again?

Terrific. Turn the page, and let's get reacquainted with some old friends.

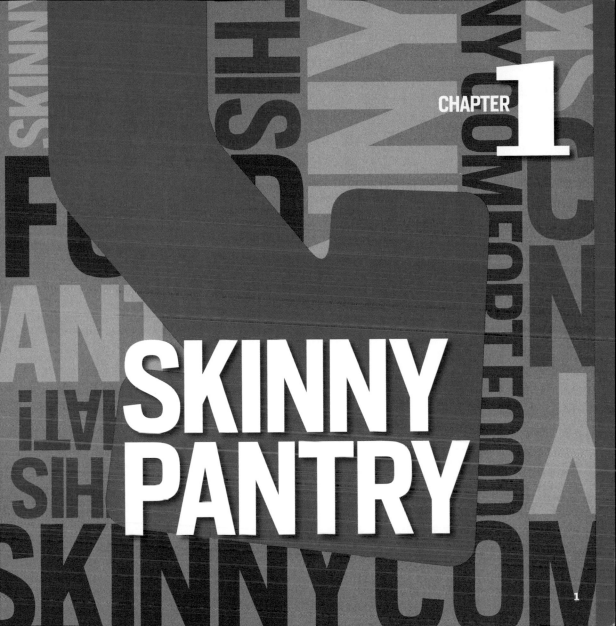

CHAPTER 1

SKINNY PANTRY

If you want to make great comfort food, you've got to do one thing first:

Get comfortable.

GET COMFORTABLE IN YOUR KITCHEN.
Get comfortable in the supermarket.
Get comfortable wielding pots and pans,
stocking your fridge and pantry, making
smart decisions in the grocery aisles.

Nowadays, most of us are more
comfortable shouting "cheeseburger with
fries" into a squawk box from our car
window than we are making a cheeseburger
and fries in our own kitchens. Whereas once
the fridge was the starting place for every
meal, now it's the ending place—a sad,
chilly refuge for forgotten takeout leftovers
slowly morphing into epic fungal art
projects. Whereas once the kitchen was
the very center of the home, nowadays it's
just a small patch of linoleum we have to
venture into in order to get ice cubes.

It's time to rethink the kitchen. Instead
of a forbidding dungeon where things get
beaten, shredded, and burned, it needs to

become the safest room in the house.
It needs to become your Bat Cave, your
Cone of Silence, your base camp at the
bottom of Everest—the place you can retreat
to for safety, for comfort, to gather up the
tools you need for your next great adventure.

Because that's what a kitchen really
should be: the base camp of life. Eating
well, feeling nourished, and staying fit and
healthy are hard jobs out there in the real
world. Your kitchen is your green zone.

So in this chapter, we've created
a complete inventory of all the tools and
foods you'll need to create the ultimate
Skinny Kitchen. Most of them you'll
already have on hand. Others you'll need
to stock up on. But knowing you have
the absolute best tools on hand will give
you the confidence you need to whip up
the many simple recipes in this book.
Ready to get comfortable?

The Skinny Pantry

The 50 best staples for building healthy, flavorful meals any time of the day.

Choosing between mayonnaises and canned tomatoes might seem like trivial stuff, but the health implications can be massive. Make just two swaps that save you 100 calories a day and you stand to lose 10 pounds in a year. We've laid out the purest, healthiest, most delicious staples to pack into your pantry. Consider these the building blocks not just for amazing comfort classics, but for a lifetime of leanness.

1. BUTTER

Eat This

Land O Lakes Unsalted Whipped Butter (1 Tbsp)
50 calories
6 g fat (3.5 g saturated)
0 mg sodium

By using whipped butter, you can enjoy the taste of real butter for half the calories.

Not That!

Imperial Vegetable Oil Spread (1 Tbsp)
70 calories
7 g fat
(1.5 g saturated, 1.5 g trans)
105 mg sodium

This margarine contains the absolute maximum amount of trans fat you should consume within a day in every tablespoon.

2. OIL

Eat This

Pure Wesson 100% Natural Canola Oil (1 Tbsp)
120 calories
14 g fat (1 g saturated)
Canola boasts a near-perfect ratio of omega-6 to omega-3 fats, making it an ideal all-purpose oil for sautéing, roasting, and making dressings.

Not That!

Crisco Pure Vegetable Oil (1 Tbsp)
120 calories
14 g fat (2 g saturated)
Soybean oil—which is what Crisco uses—is low in heart-friendly monounsaturated fats.

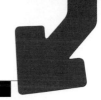

3. FLOUR

Eat This

King Arthur Unbleached White Whole Wheat Flour
(¼ cup)
100 calories
0.5 g fat
3 g fiber

This flour combines the fiber of wheat with a taste and texture similar to regular white flour.

Not That!

Gold Medal All-Purpose Flour
(¼ cup)
100 calories
0 g fat
<1 g fiber

All flour starts out full of fiber, but nearly all of it is lost in the refining process.

4. ORANGE JUICE

Drink This

Tropicana Trop50 Some Pulp
(8 fl oz)
50 calories
0 g fat
10 g sugars

Trop50 is partially sweetened by Purevia, which helps to cut down on sugars.

Not That!

SunnyD Tangy Original
(8 fl oz)
60 calories
0 g fat
14 g sugars

SunnyD contains 5 percent orange juice. The other 95 percent? High fructose corn syrup, oil, and a host of other low-grade additives.

5. SLICED BREAD

Eat This

Arnold Healthfull 10 Multigrain (1 slice)
45 calories
0.5 g fat (0 g saturated)
85 mg sodium
4 g fiber

This bread may be two grains down, but packs double the fiber per slice.

Not That!

Nature's Pride 12-Grain Bread (1 slice)
110 calories
2 g fat (0 g saturated)
150 mg sodium
2 g fiber

This slice is one of the most calorie-dense breads in the supermarket. Too bad it doesn't have the fiber to justify the high caloric cost.

6. HAMBURGER BUNS

Eat This

Martin's Potato Rolls
(1 bun)
130 calories
1.5 g fat (0 g saturated)
200 mg sodium
3 g fiber

We love that these rolls pack 3 grams of fiber into 130 calories, but we also love that Martin's is the bun of choice for many of the country's burger masters.

Not That!

Arnold Select Hamburger Rolls
(1 bun)
160 calories
2 g fat (0 g saturated)
250 mg sodium

Each bun is more caloric than a McDonald's hamburger patty.

The Skinny Pantry

7. ENGLISH MUFFINS

Eat This

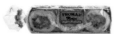

Thomas' Light Multi-Grain English Muffins (1 muffin)
100 calories
1 g fat (0 g saturated)
26 g carbohydrates
160 mg sodium

Thomas' manages to cram 8 grams of fiber—that's as much as a Fiber One bar!—into every muffin.

Not That!

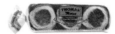

Thomas' Honey Wheat English Muffins (1 muffin)
130 calories
0.5 g fat (0 g saturated)
26 g carbohydrates
190 mg sodium

One gram of fiber is a waste of a muffin.

8. TORTILLAS

Eat This

Mission White Corn Tortillas (2)
90 calories
1 g fat (0 g saturated)
10 g sodium
3 g fiber

Corn tortillas actually count as a whole-grain option, since they're made with whole corn kernels, water, and little else.

Not That!

Mission Flour Tortillas, small (2)
220 calories
5 g fat (2 g saturated)
620 mg sodium
2 g fiber

Flour tortillas lose to corn in every major category: calories, fat, sodium, carbs, fiber, and number of ingredients.

9. WHOLE-WHEAT TORTILLAS

Eat This

La Tortilla Factory Smart & Delicious Low Carb High Fiber Large Tortilla (1)
80 calories
3 g fat (0 g saturated)
300 mg sodium
12 g fiber

One tortilla supplies half of the daily fiber requirement for women (and nearly half for men).

Not That!

Mission Multi-Grain Medium Tortilla (1)
150 calories
4 g fat (1.5 g saturated)
310 mg sodium
5 g fiber

Five grams of fiber isn't bad, but you can do a lot better for 150 calories.

10. PASTA

Eat This

Ronzoni Smart Taste Elbows (2 oz dry)
170 calories
0.5 g fat (0 g saturated)
5 g fiber

The best of both worlds: the familiar taste of traditional pasta, but with 5 grams of fiber and 40 fewer calories per serving. Make this your go-to pasta.

Not That!

Ronzoni Elbows (2 oz dry)
210 calories
1 g fat (0 g saturated)
2 g fiber

Consuming fiber with pasta is vital as it will help keep your blood sugar stable as you take in the crush of carbs. Two grams per serving, though, is just not going to cut it.

11. GRAINS

Eat This

Bob's Red Mill Organic Whole Grain Quinoa
(¼ cup dry)
170 calories
2.5 g fat (0 g saturated)
4 g fiber

Quinoa is a complete protein—It contains every amino acid needed for proper nutrition. Add 4 grams of fiber per serving, and it's the ultimate meal base.

Not That!

Near East Pearled Couscous Original Plain
(⅓ cup dry, as packaged)
210 calories
0 g fat
2 g fiber

Couscous is more pasta than whole grain, which explains the low fiber count.

12. PILAF

Eat This

Near East Wheat Pilaf
(1 cup prepared)
200 calories
4.5 g fat (2 g saturated)
680 mg sodium
8 g fiber

With 8 grams of fiber in every cup, this bulgur-based pilaf packs more than double the amount found in brown rice.

Not That!

Rice-A-Roni Rice Pilaf
(1 cup prepared)
310 calories
9 g fat
(1.5 g saturated, 1.5 g trans)
1,060 mg sodium
2 g fiber

A cup swallows up more than two-thirds of a day's allotment of sodium and nearly a full day's worth of nasty trans fats.

13. RICE

Eat This

Lundberg Long Grain Brown Rice (¼ cup dry)
150 calories
1.5 g fat (0 g saturated)
3 g fiber

If you're going to make rice a part of your meal regimen, make sure it has at least 3 grams of fiber per serving.

Not That!

Carolina Brown Rice Whole Grain (¼ cup dry)
150 calories
1 g fat (0 g saturated)
1 g fiber

A "whole grain" that is nearly fiber-free sounds like an oxymoron, but nothing surprises us in the food world. Rice can be one of the most dangerous foods in the pantry.

14. HOT CEREAL

Eat This

Bob's Red Mill 7 Grain Hot Cereal (¼ cup dry)
140 calories
1.5 g fat (0 g saturated)
6 g fiber

Bob is a hero of the American food chain, responsible for putting out the best grains you'll find in the supermarket. This cereal is like waking up to a bowl of rocket fuel.

Not That!

Cream of Wheat Instant Original
(¼ cup dry)
160 calories
0 g fat
1 g fiber

Even a bowl of Froot Loops packs more fiber than this classic breakfast cereal. Time to find a new beginning to the day.

The Skinny Pantry

15. BISCUITS

Eat This

Pillsbury Simply Buttermilk Biscuits
(1 biscuit)
100 calories
3 g fat (1.5 g saturated)
330 mg sodium

With just 100 calories and zero trans fats, you won't find a better biscuit in the supermarket. Stuff with scrambled eggs for a breakfast bonanza.

Not That!

Alexia Biscuits
(1 biscuit)
190 calories
9 g fat (5 g saturated)
420 mg sodium

These biscuits are made with palm oil, which research has indicated promotes heart disease.

16. CRACKERS

Eat This

Triscuits
(6 crackers)
120 calories
4 g fat (1 g saturated)
140 mg sodium
3 g fiber

Our favorite cracker of all time, not just because it has 3 grams of fiber, but because it pairs with everything from Cheddar to chocolate to salsa.

Not That!

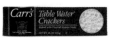

Carr's Table Water Crackers
(8 crackers)
120 calories
2 g fat (0 g saturated)
130 mg sodium
0 g fiber

A fiber-free cracker is only a small step above a cookie.

17. CHICKEN STOCK

Eat This

Kitchen Basics Original Chicken Stock
(1 cup)
20 calories
0 g fat
430 mg sodium

Stocks are less seasoned (read: less salty) than broths so as to let other ingredients' flavors come through. Good for your food; good for your body.

Not That!

College Inn Chicken Broth
(1 cup)
15 calories
1 g fat (0 g saturated)
930 mg sodium

Both neurotoxin MSG and partially hydrogenated oil, the source of trans fats, plague this broth.

18. BEEF STOCK

Eat This

Swanson Unsalted 100% Natural Beef Flavored Stock
(1 cup)
20 calories
0 g fat
140 mg sodium

Swanson's regular stock contains 350 percent more sodium than the unsalted version.

Not That!

Emeril's All Natural Beef Flavored Stock
(1 cup)
15 calories
0 g fat
630 mg sodium

With so much sodium in the stock, it becomes impossible to control the seasoning in the soups, stews, and sauces you add it to.

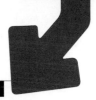

19. TOMATO SOUP

Eat This

Imagine Organic Creamy Tomato Soup
(1 cup)
80 calories
1 g fat
620 mg sodium
2 g fiber

A study found that organic tomatoes contain nearly double the amount of flavonoid antioxidants than conventional crops.

Not That!

Campbell's Slow Kettle Style Soups Tomato & Sweet Basil Bisque
(1 cup)
260 calories
14 g fat (8 g saturated)
750 mg sodium
3 g fiber

This bisque packs as much fat as two scoops of Edy's Grand Mud Pie ice cream.

20. BAKED BEANS

Eat This

Bush's Best Baked Beans Maple Cured Bacon (½ cup)
140 calories
1 g fat (0 g saturated)
620 mg sodium
5 g fiber

Baked beans in general rely too heavily on sugar, but at least these are bolstered by a potent combination of fiber and protein.

Not That!

B&M Baked Beans Bacon & Onion
(½ cup)
190 calories
2 g fat (0.5 g saturated)
450 mg sodium
8 g fiber

There are five different sources of sugar listed on the ingredient statement.

21. REFRIED BEANS

Eat This

Eden Organic Refried Pinto Beans
(½ cup)
90 calories
1 g fat (0 g saturated)
180 mg sodium
7 g fiber

Not just an excellent source of protein and fiber, beans are also loaded with anthocyanins, antioxidants that help fight off disease.

Not That!

Ortega Refried Beans
(⅓ cup)
150 calories
2.5 g fat (1 g saturated)
570 mg sodium
9 g fiber

The benefits of beans are undercut here by a bit too much oil and way too much salt.

22. TOMATOES

Eat This

San Marzano Crushed Tomatoes (½ cup)
40 calories
0 g fat
190 mg sodium

San Marzano tomatoes are considered by many to naturally be the best, sweetest sauce base in the world. No need for excess sugar and salt in these cans.

Not That!

Del Monte Stewed Tomatoes Mexican Recipe (½ cup)
40 calories
0 g fat
340 mg sodium

Salt is fourth on the ingredient statement, and just 1 serving contains 20 percent of your entire day's sodium allotment.

The Skinny Pantry

23. MARINARA SAUCE

Eat This

Lidia's Marinara
(½ cup)
60 calories
2 g fat (0 g saturated)
350 mg sodium

Lidia Bastianich is one of the great pioneers of Italian cooking in America and her sauces reflect her culinary philosophy: first-rate ingredients messed with as little as possible.

Not That!

De Cecco Marinara
(½ cup)
80 calories
2.5 g fat (0 g saturated)
680 mg sodium

More calories, fat, sugar, and total ingredients than Lidia's. Plus, 1 serving knocks out nearly half of your daily sodium allotment.

24. PESTO

Eat This

Sacla Italia Sun Dried Tomato & Garlic Pesto Sauce (¼ cup)
110 calories
10 g fat (1 g saturated)
340 mg sodium

With healthy sun-dried tomatoes as the primary ingredient powering this pesto, there's less room for oil to drive up the calorie count.

Not That!

Mezzetta Homemade Style Basil Pesto
(¼ cup)
300 calories
32 g fat (5 g saturated)
640 mg sodium

This sauce harbors more fat than a bacon-topped Double Stacker from Burger King.

25. JELLY

Eat This

Smuckers Simply Fruit Blueberry
(1 Tbsp)
40 calories
0 g fat
8 g sugars

The mark of a great jam is being 100 percent fruit. Smuckers makes this fantastic line with nothing but fruit and fruit juice concentrates.

Not That!

Welch's Concord Grape Jam (1 Tbsp)
50 calories
0 g fat
13 g sugars

Sometimes the most vital facts lie in the ingredient statement. There you'll find that corn syrup and high-fructose corn syrup are the second and third ingredients in this spread.

26. FRUIT PRESERVES

Eat This

Medford Farms Apple Butter
(1 Tbsp)
25 calories
0 g fat
4 g sugars

This sweet spread is made purely from apples. Try it on toast, drizzled on ice cream, or spread on a warm biscuit.

Not That!

Smuckers Sweet Orange Marmalade
(1 Tbsp)
50 calories
0 g fat
12 g sugars

The first two ingredients are high-fructose corn syrup and corn syrup.

27. SYRUP

Eat This

**Maple Grove Farms
100% Pure Maple
Syrup Dark Amber**
(¼ cup)

*200 calories
0 g fat
53 g sugars*

Real maple syrup is a top
source of manganese and
zinc—both important
immune system boosters.

Not That!

**Eggo
Original Syrup**
(¼ cup)

*240 calories
0 g fat
40 g sugars*

This syrup is packed
with more calories than the
waffles it tops, and
all of them are supplied by
refined sugars.

28. PEANUT BUTTER

Eat This

**Justin's Classic
Almond Butter** (2 Tbsp)

*200 calories
18 g fat (2 g saturated)
0 mg sodium*

New research indicates
that almond-derived
calories may not be fully
absorbed by our bodies,
which gives us even more
reason to love this sweet,
creamy spread.

Not That!

Jif Natural Creamy
(2 Tbsp)

*190 calories
16 g fat (3 g saturated)
80 mg sodium*

This "natural" spread
is rife with added sugars
and palm oil. The best
peanut butters have
two ingredients: peanuts
and salt.

29. BARBECUE SAUCE

Eat This

**Stubb's
Bar-B-Q Sauce
Mild** (2 Tbsp)

*25 calories
0 g fat
230 mg sodium*

This tomato-based
sauce gets its flavorful kick
from a blend of antioxidant-
rich spices.

Not That!

**Kraft Original
Barbecue Sauce**
(2 Tbsp)

*50 calories
0 g fat
270 mg sodium*

Two tablespoons of this
sauce contain as much
sugar as an entire bowl of
Lucky Charms cereal.

30. SPICY CHILI SAUCE

Eat This

Huy Fong Sriracha
(1 Tbsp)

*15 calories
0 g fat
300 mg sodium*

Capsaicin, the compound
that gives chiles their heat,
is known to increase
metabolism. This sauce,
made almost entirely from
chiles, will kick your fat-
burning engine into full gear.

Not That!

**Asian Gourmet
Chili Oil** (1 Tbsp)

*130 calories
14 g fat (3 g saturated)
0 mg sodium*

You'll find this condiment
on tables in restaurants
across Asia (and
increasingly in America,
too). There are lighter,
more concentrated ways to
get your spicy fix.

The Skinny Pantry

31. MAYONNAISE

Eat This

**Kraft Mayo
with Olive Oil
Reduced Fat
Mayonnaise (1 Tbsp)**
*45 calories
4 g fat (0 g saturated)
95 mg sodium*

The olive oil in this mayo supplies polyphenols, antioxidants that help your body ward off disease.

Not That!

**Hellmann's
Real Mayonnaise
(1 Tbsp)**
*90 calories
10 g fat (1.5 g saturated)
90 mg sodium*

If a magical mayo with half the calories of your normal spread existed, why wouldn't you use it?

32. SALSA

Eat This

**Muir Glen
Organic Garlic
Cilantro Salsa
(2 Tbsp)**
*10 calories
0 g fat
130 mg sodium*

The Muir Glen ingredient list reads like a stroll through an organic garden.

Not That!

**Tostitos
Restaurant Style Salsa
(2 Tbsp)**
*15 calories
0 g fat
210 mg sodium*

Salt is listed as the first seasoning in this salsa.

33. GUACAMOLE

Eat This

**Wholly Guacamole
Classic
(2 Tbsp)**
*60 calories
5 g fat (1 g saturated)
90 mg sodium*

The closest thing to homemade guacamole you're going to find in the supermarket.

Not That!

**Mission Guacamole
Flavored Dip
(2 Tbsp)**
*40 calories
3 g fat (0 g saturated)
150 mg sodium*

Oil, cornstarch, and "avocado powder" replace real avocados in this guacamole imposter.

34. RANCH DRESSING

Eat This

**Bolthouse Farms
Classic Ranch (2 Tbsp)**
*45 calories
3 g fat (0.5 g saturated)
270 mg sodium*

Ranch, one of the highest-calorie condiments on the planet, is normally nothing but trouble, but Bolthouse uses a yogurt base to give this dressing creaminess without the fat.

Not That!

**Hidden Valley
The Original Ranch
(2 Tbsp)**
*140 calories
14 g fat (2.5 g saturated)
260 mg sodium*

Two spoonfuls of this dressing pack as much fat as a Taco Bell Beef Gordita Supreme.

35. VINAIGRETTE

Eat This

**Marie's
Balsamic Vinaigrette**
(2 Tbsp)
*50 calories
4.5 g fat (0.5 g saturated)
210 mg sodium*

Balsamic and red wine
vinegars supply flavor
without adding too many
calories. A fantastic all-
purpose dressing to keep
around for your salad needs.

Not That!

**Newman's Own Olive
Oil & Vinegar Dressing**
(2 Tbsp)
*150 calories
16 g fat (2.5 g saturated)
150 mg sodium*

Newman sticks to
a more traditional
3-to-1 oil-to-vinegar ratio,
which gives this dressing
its caloric heft.

36. SOY SAUCE

Eat This

**Kikkoman
Less Sodium
Soy Sauce**
(1 Tbsp)
*10 calories
0 g fat
575 mg sodium*

A solid choice to keep in
your pantry for stir-fries
and marinades. Even with
the sodium reduction,
apply this sauce sparingly.

Not That!

**La Choy
Soy Sauce**
(1 Tbsp)
*10 calories
0 g fat
1,160 mg sodium*

Each tablespoon packs
more sodium than an
entire can of Pringles.
Stock your pantry with this
at your own peril.

37. ASIAN SAUCE

Eat This

**La Choy
Teriyaki Stir Fry Sauce**
(1 Tbsp)
*10 calories
0 g fat
105 mg sodium*

This sauce manages to
avoid the two most
common pitfalls of Asian
condiments: excess sodium
and excess sugars.

Not That!

**House of Tsang Saigon
Sizzle Stir-Fry Sauce**
(1 Tbsp)
*45 calories
2 g fat (0 g saturated)
380 mg sodium*

A single tablespoon
holds as much sugar
as two Keebler Fudge
Stripes cookies.

38. CRUMBLED CHEESE

Eat This

**President
Crumbled Feta** (1 oz)
*70 calories
5 g fat (3.5 g saturated)
260 mg sodium*

Feta's full, pungent flavor
belies a surprisingly low
caloric tax. Try mixing with
chopped olives, tomatoes,
garlic, and basil for an
incredible salsa for grilled
chicken or steak.

Not That!

**Alouette
Blue Cheese**
(1 oz)
*100 calories
8 g fat (5 g saturated)
260 mg sodium*

Blue cheese is among
the most caloric of the
crumbled cheeses.

The Skinny Pantry

39. SHREDDED CHEESE

Eat This

Kraft Shredded Low-Moisture Part-Skim Mozzarella (¼ cup)

70 calories
5 g fat (3 g saturated)
180 mg sodium

Consider part-skim dairy products a more flavorful, less rubbery medium between "low fat" and "full fat."

Not That!

Kraft Natural Cheese Shredded Sharp Cheddar Cheese (¼ cup)

110 calories
9 g fat (6 g saturated)
180 mg sodium

A quarter-cup of this three-cheese blend packs more saturated fat than two Twinkies!

40. SLICED CHEESE

Eat This

Kraft Singles 2% Milk Sharp Cheddar (1 slice)

45 calories
3 g fat (1.5 g saturated)
250 mg sodium

These slices are the key to guilt-free grilled cheese. Also one of our favorite ways to top a cheeseburger.

Not That!

Kraft Deli Deluxe Sharp Cheddar Slices (1 slice)

110 calories
9 g fat (5 g saturated)
450 mg sodium

One slice contains more saturated fat than an entire box of Kraft Mac and Cheese.

41. RICOTTA CHEESE

Eat This

Polly-O Part Skim Ricotta Cheese (¼ cup)

90 calories
6 g fat (4 g saturated)
65 mg sodium

Each quarter cup has as much protein as a glass of milk. Try adding a scoop to your next batch of mac and cheese for an extra creamy texture.

Not That!

Sorrento Whole Milk Ricotta Cheese (¼ cup)

120 calories
9 g fat (5 g saturated)
55 mg sodium

With whole milk as its base, Sorrento's ricotta packs 50 percent more fat than Polly-O's.

42. CREAM CHEESE

Eat This

Philadelphia Whipped Cream Cheese (2 Tbsp)

60 calories
5 g fat (3 g saturated)
95 mg sodium

The whipping process introduces air into the cream cheese, making it both lighter and easier to spread. That means no accidentally overloading your breakfast breads.

Not That!

Organic Valley Organic Regular Cream Cheese (2 Tbsp)

100 calories
10 g fat (6 g saturated)
100 mg sodium

Organic saturated fat is still saturated fat, and two spoonfuls of this spread pack 30 percent of your daily max.

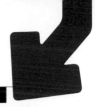

43. TUNA

Eat This

Wild Planet Wild Skipjack Light Tuna
(2 oz)
69 calories
2 g fat (0.7 g saturated)
268 mg sodium

In addition to being sustainable and packed in BPA-free cans, Wild Planet's tuna contains more omega-3 fatty acids and less mercury.

Not That!

Starkist Solid White Albacore in Vegetable Oil
(2 oz)
90 calories
4 g fat (1 g saturated)
210 mg sodium

Conventional albacore contains about three times as much mercury as light tuna.

44. DELI MEAT

Eat This

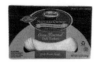

Hormel Natural Choice Oven Roasted Deli Turkey (56 g)
60 calories
1 g fat (0 g saturated)
460 mg sodium
11 g protein

More protein, fewer calories, and no added nitrates? Sign us up!

Not That!

Land O'Frost Premium Oven Roasted Turkey Breast (50 g)
70 calories
3 g fat (1 g saturated)
560 mg sodium
9 g protein

Proof that not all turkey meat is necessarily lean.

45. BACON

Eat This

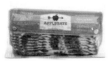

Applegate Naturals Sunday Bacon
(2 strips, 14 g)
60 calories
5 g fat (2 g saturated)
290 mg sodium

Not only is this as lean and meaty as bacon gets, Applegate also avoids using potentially harmful nitrites when curing this pork.

Not That!

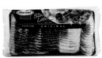

Hormel Black Label Maple
(2 strips, 18 g)
90 calories
7 g fat (2.5 g saturated)
310 mg sodium

This bacon contains sodium nitrite and caramel coloring, both of which are linked to cancer.

46. ITALIAN SAUSAGE

Eat This

Aidells Italian Style with Mozzarella Cheese
(1 link, 85 g)
170 calories
12 g fat (3.5 g saturated)
580 mg sodium

Aidells keeps the fat count down by using only mozzarella, a naturally lighter cheese.

Not That!

Hillshire Farm Gourmet Creations Sweet Italian Style with Peppers and Mozzarella Cheese
(1 link, 84 g)
280 calories
24 g fat (9 g saturated)
580 mg sodium

More calories and fat, and less protein than Aidells.

The Skinny Pantry

47. CHICKEN SAUSAGE

Eat This

Applegate Organics Chicken & Apple Chicken Sausage
(1 link, 85 g)
140 calories
7 g fat (1.5 g saturated)
500 mg sodium

The top two ingredients are chicken and dried apples. A perfect example of why we love all of Applegate's products so much.

Not That!

Johnsonville Chicken Sausage Apple
(1 link, 85 g)
180 calories
12 g fat (2.5 g saturated)
820 mg sodium

Chicken, water, and corn syrup dominate the ingredient statement. What makes up less than 2 percent? Apples.

48. HOT DOGS

Eat This

Applegate The Great Organic Original Beef Hot Dog
(1 link, 48 g)
90 calories
6 g fat (2.5 g saturated)
380 mg sodium

Applegate's dogs are made from grass-fed beef, which has a higher concentration of healthy fats.

Not That!

Ball Park Jumbo Beef Franks
(1 link)
240 calories
20 g fat
(8 g saturated, 1 g trans)
670 mg sodium

Between the trans fats and the precipitous sodium count, these are some dangerous dogs.

49. FRENCH FRIES

Eat This

Cascadian Farm Shoe String French Fries
(85 g)
110 calories
5 g fat (1 g saturated)
10 mg sodium

Cascadian Farm lightly brushes its fries with pure canola oil, which gives them a crisp exterior without soaking them in excess calories.

Not That!

McCain 5 Minute Fries
(85 g)
200 calories
8 g fat (1 g saturated)
220 mg sodium

These fries are doused in an oil blend which saddles them with as many calories as real french fries.

50. ICE CREAM

Eat This

Breyers Natural Vanilla (½ cup)
130 calories
7 g fat (4 g saturated)
14 g sugars

Breyers uses more milk than cream, helping to keep this ice cream commendably light. Make this line your standard choice for sundaes, milk shakes, and midnight carton raiding.

Not That!

SheerBliss Vanilla (½ cup)
300 calories
19 g fat (13 g saturated)
27 g sugars

Move over, Häagen-Dazs. This new line of so-called premium ice cream manages to cram even more fat and sugar into its pints.

10 BEST Supermarket Comfort Foods

The healthiest ways to bring comfort to your kitchen when there's not enough time to do it yourself.

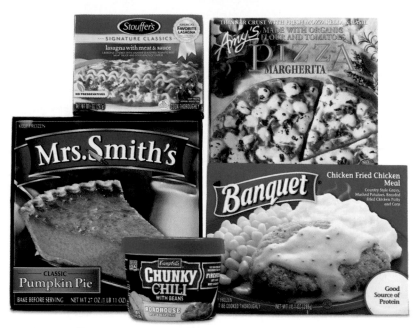

1. LASAGNA
Stouffer's Lasagna with Meat & Sauce
(1 package, 297 g)

340 calories
12 g fat
(6 g saturated,
0.5 g trans)
850 mg sodium
This traditional favorite is also surprisingly moderate, thanks to judicious use of part-skim mozzarella and fat-free milk and cottage cheese.

2. PIE
Mrs. Smith's Pumpkin Pie
(⅛ pie, 127 g)

280 calories
14 g fat
(6 g saturated)
17 g sugars
Pumpkin is rich in vision-boosting vitamin A, and just one slice of this pie fulfills 45 percent of your recommended daily value.

3. CHILI
Campbell's Chunky Roadhouse Chili (1 cup)

220 calories
6 g fat
(3 g saturated)
870 mg sodium
One cup contains less fat, more fiber, more protein, and fewer calories than an entire Baked Chicken Lean Cuisine frozen meal. Top with diced raw onions and a shake of hot sauce.

4. PIZZA
Amy's Single Serve Margherita Pizza
(1 pizza, 176 g)

400 calories
17 g fat
(5 g saturated)
720 mg sodium
A fantastic alternative to delivery. Dress it up with fresh produce, turkey pepperoni, or chicken sausage.

5. FRIED CHICKEN
Banquet Chicken Fried Chicken Meal (1 entrée, 286 g)

350 calories
17 g fat
(4 g saturated)
930 mg sodium
A complete meal of chicken, corn, and mashed potatoes, all for fewer calories than you'd find in two Outback Steakhouse hot wings.

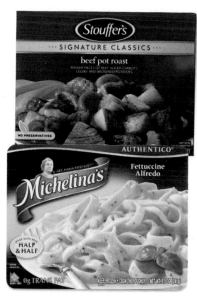
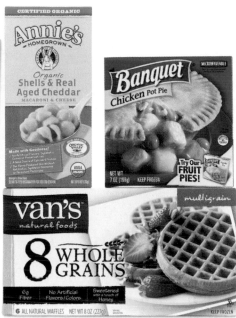

6. POT ROAST
Stouffer's Beef Pot Roast
(1 package, 251 g)

230 calories
7 g fat
(2 g saturated)
820 mg sodium
Stouffer's specializes in comfort food, and many of their dishes are impressively low in calories. Serve this beefy blend atop quinoa for a hunger-quashing meal.

7. ALFREDO
Michelina's Authentic Fettuccine Alfredo
(1 package, 241 g)

310 calories
10 g fat
(6 g saturated)
650 mg sodium
Michelina's uses half-and-half instead of heavy cream to create the lightest Alfredo we've seen anywhere.

8. MAC & CHEESE
Annie's Organic Shells & Real Aged Cheddar
(1 cup prepared)

280 calories
4.5 g fat
(2.5 g saturated)
520 mg sodium
The two main ingredients are pasta and organic cheese—no FrankIngredients to be found. Power-up the pasta with ham, steamed broccoli, and sun-dried tomatoes.

9. POT PIE
Banquet Chicken Pot Pie (1 pie, 198 g)

400 calories
23 g fat
(8 g saturated)
780 mg sodium
Banquet is one of the few pot pie manufacturers that doesn't try to disguise one pie as two servings. Consider this one of the only pot pies safe enough to eat (besides our own—on page 190—of course).

10. WAFFLES
Van's 8 Whole Grains Multi-grain Waffles
(2 waffles, 76 g)

160 calories
6 g fat
(0 g saturated)
230 mg sodium
6 g fiber
These fiber-rich waffles are made from quinoa, amaranth, and millet flours. Cover with a bit of peanut butter, sliced banana, and a drizzle of agave syrup.

The A-Team

These powerful pantry players are the key to cooking dishes that are both intensely flavorful and incredibly lean.

Agave Syrup

Made from the same form of blue agave used to produce tequila, agave syrup is sweeter than sugar (about 1.5 times sweeter) yet has a very low glycemic index. Debate is ongoing, but many scientists believe that sweetening foods with agave syrup may have a gentler impact on your blood sugar than sugar, which is exactly what you want, since those spikes both deplete you of energy and signal your body to start storing fat. This natural sweetener has just the taste and the texture to fit seamlessly into most recipes in this book.
How to Use It: As a substitute for maple syrup on pancakes and waffles; as a sweetener for iced tea, coffee, and cocktails; to flavor unsweetened yogurt or oatmeal; in any savory recipe in this book that calls for sugar.

2% Milk

In most professional kitchens, heavy cream is as common a staple ingredient as salt and pepper. Not only does that spell doom for your waistline, but it also gives food a uniformly heavy, fatty feel that leaves little room for other flavors. That's why we love milk: it lends a bit of dairy creaminess to soups, sauces, and desserts without muscling out the real stars of the recipe. Why 2%? Because some of milk's best nutrients are fat soluble, meaning your body needs a bit of fat to fully absorb them. Plus, a little fat can be a lovely thing.
How to Use It: Use to make béchamel, which forms the base for mac and cheese, pot pie, and lasagna; stir into chowders; in recipes that call for heavy cream, try using three parts 2% milk to one part Greek yogurt as a low-calorie substitute.

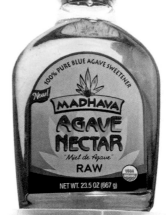

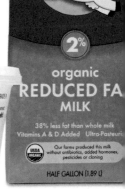

Greek Yogurt

The Greeks have had thousands of years to perfect yogurt. By skimming off the watery whey from the milk, you get a final product that packs twice as much protein as standard yogurt. More than that, you also get a yogurt with an intensely rich, creamy texture that works in both sweet and savory dishes.

How to Use It: Mix with chopped garlic, lemon juice, olive oil, and fresh herbs to make a sauce for lamb, steak, or grilled fish; scoop it onto tacos or baked potatoes as a replacement for sour cream; stir into sauces or soups instead of heavy cream.

Canned Whole Peeled Tomatoes

The little-known secret behind most great Italian restaurants' red sauce is that it's made with canned tomatoes. That's because canned tomatoes are picked at the height of the tomato season and canned instantly, preserving the intensely sweet, acidic flavor of summer tomatoes. We love whole peeled tomatoes more than, say, diced or crushed tomatoes because they're minimally processed, giving you a fresher-tasting final product. Muir Glen makes our favorite tomato products.

How to Use It: Use it as the base for homemade salsa; combine the tomatoes with nothing more than olive oil and salt for a perfect pizza sauce; use as the base for a slow-cooked dish, like our Provençal Chicken on page 178; make the perfect pasta sauce by simmering with onions, garlic, and chili flakes sautéed in olive oil

Chicken Stock

Restaurants typically use butter and cream as the base for most of their sauces, which explains a lot about why restaurant food is so disastrous to your waistline. Using chicken stock—to moisten stuffing, to build sauces, to braise meat and vegetables—gives you the flavors of roasted chicken and root vegetables with minimal caloric impact (about 10 per ½ cup). Of course, vegetable and beef stock are both excellent, but for our money, chicken is the most flavorful and the most versatile. Learn how to make your own on page 96.

How to Use It: Combine with equal parts red or white wine, plus shallots and herbs, and boil until reduced to sauce consistency (perfect for steak or chicken); stretch a pasta sauce without boosting calories by adding a few splashes of stock; deglaze a skillet or a roasting pan you cooked meat in with a cup of stock, then add a few pinches of flour and a pat of butter for instant gravy.

Balsamic Vinegar

Balsamic is probably the most famous vinegar of all, beloved for its tangy-sweet taste. Granted, real balsamic from Italy must be aged a minimum of 12 years in multiple barrels, but who's counting? The supermarket standard is still perfect as a base for building salad dressings and marinades, as well as a special secret touch when caramelizing onions, braising meat in a slow cooker, or quick-pickling vegetables.

How to Use It: Combine with equal parts soy sauce, plus chopped garlic, for a great steak or chicken marinade; mix with two parts olive oil, a small spoonful of Dijon, and salt and pepper for an all-purpose vinaigrette; cover onions or cucumbers with balsamic for 10 minutes for an instant pickle; combine with chopped strawberries and pour over vanilla ice cream (trust us!).

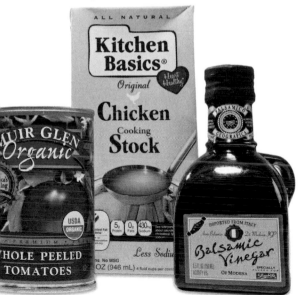

Anatomy of a Dietary Disaster

How five comfort classics go wrong,
and how you can rescue them in your own kitchen.

It's a cruel reality that the most comforting food is so often the most damaging to our bodies. Salt, sugar, fat: These form the basis of so many of our collective cravings, as well as the framework behind so many of America's greatest health problems. After spending months in the kitchen running through the full gamut of comfort foods, we've learned a lot about the perils of the most familiar foods in America, especially when left to the devices of corporate kitchens looking to maximize profit.

    To help ensure that comfort food and healthy food aren't mutually exclusive, we've done a full autopsy on five of the most iconic American comfort dishes, pinpointing the major trouble spots and offering quick, easy-to-adapt fixes for each. The tricks and techniques on the pages to come are not just meant to right the nutritional wrongs of these specific dishes, but to serve as a blueprint for keeping all your favorite comfort foods comfortably lean.

1. MAC & CHEESE

Look up "comfort food" in a dictionary and you'll see a bubbling crock of mac and cheese. Problem is, short of eating mayonnaise straight from the jar, you'd be hard-pressed to find a food with more calories per gram than macaroni and cheese from a restaurant kitchen. But we believe that a creamy, cheesy, relatively healthy bowl of mac and cheese is an inalienable right of every American, and we think we've cracked the code.

The cheese

Most restaurants choose to use low-cost cheese-like substances of the Velveeta variety. Problem is, these cheeses are long on fat and calories and short on true cheesy flavor. The restaurants' solution, of course, is to use more cheese, inevitably drowning the pasta in a bland bath of processed junk.

THE FIX: Opt for quality over quantity. Extra-sharp Cheddar packs twice as much cheesy intensity into every calorie as the mild variety (and about four times as much as processed cheese blocks). With the strong Cheddar flavor as the base, we work in naturally low-calorie cheeses to give the sauce more body and less caloric density. Both Swiss and mozzarella are lower in calories and fat than Cheddar and are excellent melting cheeses, giving the mac that amazing stretchy-cheese quality.

The sauce

A cautionary tale: Matt used to work at a restaurant (which shall remain unnamed) that made one of the most famous mac and cheeses in Los Angeles. What made it so famous? The recipe started with a quart of heavy cream and two sticks of butter. All of that was cooked down until thick like yogurt, then hit with an astounding heap of cheese. How many bowls did they make out of this great vat of bubbling intensity? Four, each packing an estimated 2,100 calories.

THE FIX: Béchamel, a mixture of milk, flour, and butter, is a perfect lower-calorie stand-in for any recipe calling for heavy cream or excess cheese. The point of the béchamel is to provide rich, smooth texture and stretch the impact of the cheese without burdening the pasta with unnecessary calories and fat. We make ours with 2% milk (you need a bit of fat, of course) and a light hand with the butter. Simmer until the flour combines with the milk to create a thick sauce, then stir in the cheese.

The cooking

Most mac and cheese starts in the pan, then is finished in the oven for up to 30 minutes of high-temp baking. But as the sauce bubbles away, it reduces down, thickening with each passing minute it spends in the oven. To compensate, restaurants bathe their macaroni in copious amounts of cheese sauce, which means mac and cheese often resembles an orange soup as much as it does a pasta.

THE FIX: A short, high-temperature blast under the oven's broiler gives you a crunchy caramelized crust without drying out the mac. To tease out the textural contrast even more, we add a light layer of bread crumbs and grated Parmesan, both of which brown up beautifully under the heat of the broiler.

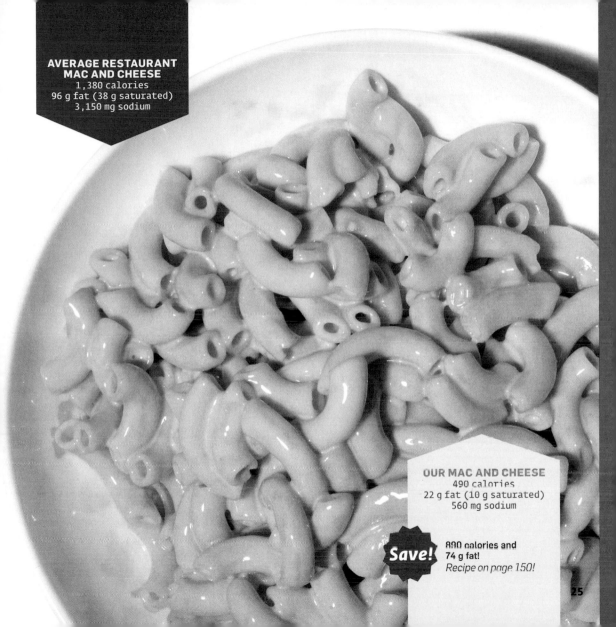

**AVERAGE RESTAURANT
MAC AND CHEESE**
1,380 calories
96 g fat (38 g saturated)
3,150 mg sodium

OUR MAC AND CHEESE
490 calories
22 g fat (10 g saturated)
560 mg sodium

Save! 890 calories and
74 g fat!
Recipe on page 150!

25

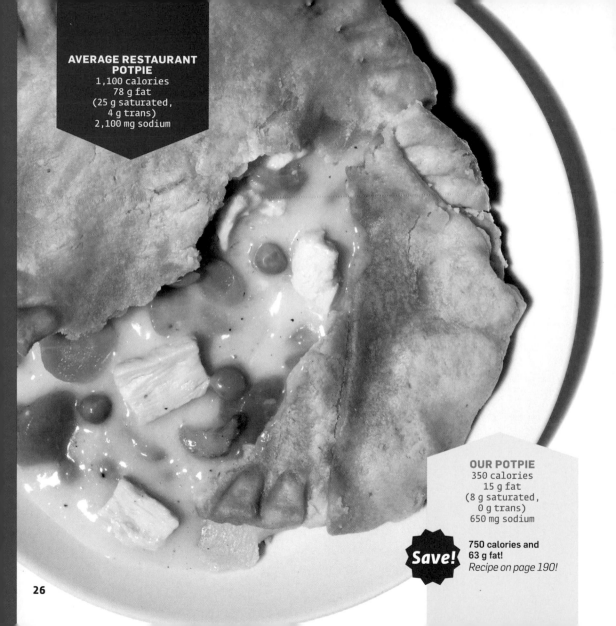

AVERAGE RESTAURANT POTPIE
1,100 calories
78 g fat
(25 g saturated,
4 g trans)
2,100 mg sodium

OUR POTPIE
350 calories
15 g fat
(8 g saturated,
0 g trans)
650 mg sodium

Save! **750 calories and 63 g fat!**
Recipe on page 190!

2. POTPIE

Potpie hits all of the touchstones of classic comfort food: It's meaty, creamy, saucy, salty, carby, and downright delicious. It's also dangerously overloaded with the kinds of ingredients that give your cardiologist nightmares: bad fats, empty carbs, sodium, low-quality calories. Of course, it doesn't have to be that way. A few simple tricks can return potpie to the realms of nutritional respectability without sacrificing the creature comforts of the original dish.

The crust

The flaky golden-brown lid may be the sexiest part of a pot-pie, but it's also the most glaring of the dish's many nutritional pitfalls. Its principle ingredients, flour and fat, pack a punch in any iteration, but the fact that shortening and other hydrogenated fats are frequently used introduces a whole new element of danger to the table: trans fats. Given that many restaurants use the pastry as both a base and a top for the potpie, you could be looking at a double dose of dietary disaster.

THE FIX: We've made really excellent potpies with phyllo dough, which gives the dish the same flaky, buttery quality with considerably fewer calories. But for those who want the full pastry effect, buy puff pastry without trans fats and use a rolling pin to stretch out the shell to a ¼-inch thickness. You will still have the buttery golden top, but for about a quarter of the calories of a standard pastry lid.

The filling

The standard potpie filling is made with heavy cream combined with butter or cheap industrial oil, cooked down until thick and gloppy. In there is a token amount of vegetables—a smattering of carrots and onions, if you're lucky—plus a big serving of dark-meat turkey or chicken.

THE FIX: Make a roux, using a small amount of oil or butter mixed with flour, chicken stock, and low-fat milk. As the flour heats up, it thickens the stock and the milk to form a creamy low-calorie base. More importantly, spike the sauce with as many vegetables you can get your hands on: Onions, carrots, potatoes, and peas should be in there of course, but other vegetables like parsnips, turnips, and mushrooms also work well. As for the meat, we prefer chunks of white-meat turkey or chicken—a pure protein addition to the potpie party.

The size

It's no secret that portion distortion is at the heart of the nutritional shortcomings of restaurant food, but dishes like potpie are particularly problematic because the size of the potpie depends entirely on the size of the serving vessel, which tends to be fabulously exaggerated. A serving of potpie should be about the size of a bowl of cereal, so think twice when the waiter shows up with a horse trough instead.

THE FIX: We prefer to make a whole batch of potpie in a single baking dish, which simplifies the cooking process and makes it easier to carve out reasonably sized individual portions. Dump the entire filling into a 13 x 9-inch baking dish, top with the pastry, and pop it into the oven.

3. STEAK AND POTATOES

Caveman steaks and overstuffed potatoes aren't just for expense account businessmen, but also for people who love the primal simplicity of a juicy cut of beef and a block of carbohydrates. It's one of the most expensive meals you can eat outside of the house—not just in terms of dollars and cents, but also calories, fat, and sodium. Here's how to cut costs across the board.

The cut

The iconic steakhouse cut, the rib eye, also happens to be among the fattiest steaks available. An 8-ounce rib eye clocks in at 554 calories and 42 grams of fat. Other popular choices don't fair much better: Porterhouse , T-bone , and tenderloin all pack 560 calories and more than 40 grams of fat per 8-ounce serving—and that's before any sauce or topping touches it.

THE FIX: We love steaks that combine big beefy flavor and maximum tenderness for minimum calories. We've run the numbers on all cuts of steak and singled out our favorites: sirloin (446 calories per 8 ounces) for being both tender and intensely meaty; flank steak (352 calories) for its pleasant chew and ability to stand up to marinades; and hanger steak (348 calories), the dark-horse winner, because no steak packs more beefiness into fewer calories.

The sauce

The classic steakhouse sauces boil down to one thing: butter. Béarnaise, hollandaise, green peppercorn—all contain lavish amounts of fat and little in the way of supporting flavors. In fact, many steakhouses don't even bother with a sauce and instead drown their beef in liberal amounts of melted butter just before serving.

THE FIX: A truly great steak needs nothing but salt and fire, but we love a great sauce as much as the next carnivore. The best route is to build around the flavor of the steak itself, combining the leftover juices and brown bits from the cooking pan with red wine and stock to create a perfect accent to the red meat. Can't imagine cooking a steak on anything other than a grill? Then serve it with a batch of chimichurri (page 319), a bright and balanced counterpoint to the char of the open flame.

The spud

A large russet potato, before a single shred of cheese or a crumb of bacon hits it, contains 290 calories, almost all of which come from quick-burning carbohydrates. Start tacking on pats of butter, scoops of sour cream, handfuls of Cheddar and that number quickly climbs above 500 calories.

THE FIX: Twice-baked potatoes may seem like a counterintuitive fix to a high-calorie problem, but hear us out: The roasted flesh of the potato is scooped out of the skin, bolstered with modest amounts of cheese, bacon, and Greek yogurt, then returned to the shell to bake until crispy and bubbling. Two large potatoes become four substantial portions, so what feels like an over-the-top indulgence is actually a savings of over 300 calories.

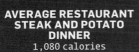

OUR STEAK AND POTATO DINNER
580 calories
28 g fat (10 g saturated)
860 mg sodium

Save! 500 calories and!
50 g fat!
Recipe on page 222!

29

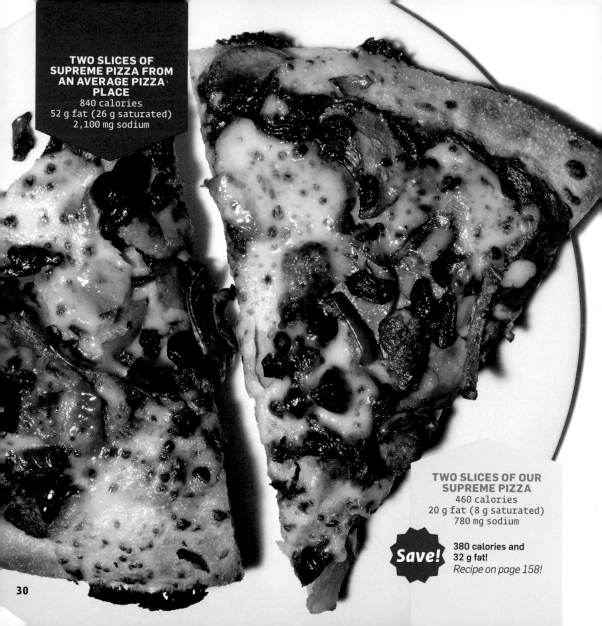

TWO SLICES OF
SUPREME PIZZA FROM
AN AVERAGE PIZZA
PLACE
840 calories
52 g fat (26 g saturated)
2,100 mg sodium

TWO SLICES OF OUR
SUPREME PIZZA
460 calories
20 g fat (8 g saturated)
780 mg sodium

Save! 380 calories and
32 g fat!
Recipe on page 158!

30

4. SUPREME PIZZA

The everything pizza, the epitome of delivery-style pie, is one governed less by the idea of balance and subtlety and more by the tried-and-true American dictum: More is more. While the nuts and bolts may vary (bacon or ham? green peppers or mushrooms?), the end result is uniformly problematic: A single slice of supreme pizza can pack more calories and saturated fat than you should consume in an entire meal. But you can have your pizza and eat it too, as long as it comes from your oven and not some delivery dude.

The toppings

A small serving of pepperoni can pack up to 140 calories. Pork sausage? About 80 calories per slice. The calories add up quickly when dealing with ingredients like this, which is why specialty pizzas from places like Domino's and Pizza Hut are so problematic to begin with.

THE FIX: Don't settle for standard pepperoni and sausage. Try Applegate Natural Pepperoni, which contains nearly half the calories and fat of the market leader, Hormel. Chicken sausage, both raw and fully cooked, from producers like Al Fresco and Aidells, should be standard replacements for all pork sausage in your kitchen, not just for pizza. Balance the meat out with plenty of nutrient-dense vegetables like mushrooms, roasted peppers, and artichoke hearts and you can turn pizza from a liability into a health boon.

The cheese

Somewhere in the chain pizza makers' handbook lies a rule that says all pizzas must be covered in a thick carpet of mediocre cheese. Low-quality mozzarella means that more is needed to actually lend flavor to the pizza, which inevitably masks the flavor of the other ingredients, the sauce, and the base of the pizza itself. It also turns a serving of pizza into a legitimate health hazard.

THE FIX: We make our pizzas with fresh mozzarella, not just because it contains fewer calories and less fat than normal packaged mozzarella, but because it actually tastes better—the creaminess is more intense, the milky awesomeness more pronounced—which means a little mozz goes a long way. Major producers like BelGioioso make high-quality fresh mozzarella on a national scale; make it a standard part of your pizza experience.

The crust

The idea of a light, airy crust is a structural impossibility with delivery pizzas for two dominant reasons: First, to support this torrent of toppings and cheese, a thicker crust is absolutely essential. Second, to survive a 20-minute ride in a cardboard box to the front door of a hungry family takes serious substance and durability. The result is a thick, chewy crust that makes up the bulk of the pizza's flavor and nutritional profile.

THE FIX: By rolling out your own dough at home, you can set the stage for a more balanced pizza. Use a rolling pin to shape thin rounds about ⅛-inch thick. If homemade dough is too daunting a task on a weekday, there are other great vessels that will work: pitas, loaves of ciabatta, and, our favorite, English muffins—which make the most perfectly sized personal pizzas imaginable.

5. ICE CREAM SUNDAE

It used to be so simple: a scoop of ice cream, a drizzle of chocolate, and a cherry on top. But those sundaes have disappeared, replaced by the mammoth creations from places like Baskin-Robbins and Cold Stone Creamery—tricked-out sundaes that contain more calories than a pound of steak and more ingredients than the most diabolical witch's brew. Follow these tips and you'll return the sundae to its rightful place as a sensible indulgence.

The ice cream

So-called premium ice creams, like those made by Häagen-Dazs, Ben & Jerry's, Cold Stone, and others, are made with heavy cream and tons of sugar, packing up to twice as many calories into a ½-cup scoop as the lighter brands out there. That means in a full-size sundae, choosing the wrong ice cream can be a difference of 300 calories or more.

THE FIX: Breyers ice cream starts not with cream but with milk. The taste and texture, though, are still spot-on. Know why? Because they don't bother with chemical fillers and other bizarre ingredients you often find in light ice creams. Breyers Natural Vanilla contains just 5 ingredients, which is exactly how it should be. If not Breyers, look for ice creams with minimal ingredients and calorie counts well below 200 per serving. Blue Bunny also fits the bill.

The toppings

Candy bars and cookies are high-calorie treats in their own right; crumbling them up and adding them to ice cream is doubling down on dessert in the worst possible way. Beyond that, beware of sneaky calories from items like peanut butter, marshmallows, and other sources of sweetness. A hundred calories of whipped cream on top of a bowl of frozen sweetened cream? There are better ways to spend calories.

THE FIX: We prefer high-impact ingredients that make an impression without saddling you with excess calories or fat. A tablespoon of dark chocolate sauce transforms a bowl of ice cream for just 50 calories. A scattering of roasted peanuts brings crunch and salty contrast for even less. And fresh fruit adds depth, natural sweetness, and a modicum of true nutrition to a dessert desperately needing some. We love to grill fruit—bananas, pineapples, peaches—because the fire adds an extra layer of flavor.

The dish

Yes, even the dish matters. Consider this study from well-known portion patroller Brian Wansink, a researcher at Cornell University. Wansink and his team invited 85 participants to an ice cream social and put out a variety of bowls and serving scoops for dishing up the dessert. The people who used large bowls and large scoops served themselves 57 percent more ice cream than those using small bowls and small scoops. The kicker? All of the participants were nutrition experts! If nutrition professors and grad students can't spot the difference, should you be expected to?

THE FIX: Yes, you can use the smallest bowl you have in the house, but an even better option is a coffee mug or a stemless wine glass, which allows you to marvel at your creation while limiting its size. Even more than the ice cream and the toppings you chose, this may be the biggest factor in determining the nutritional value of your next sundae.

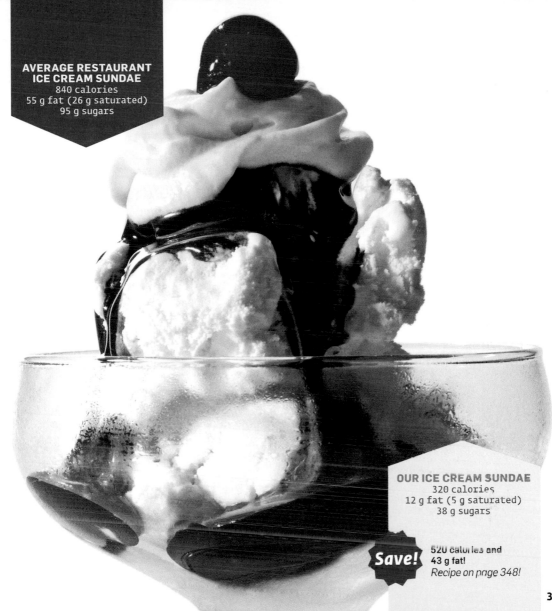

Kitchen Wisdom

The best culinary minds know that simple touches can lead to magical meals. Here are 20 kitchen tips, tricks, and philosophies that'll ensure every dish makes your taste buds happy.

1. Season to taste.

Very few of the recipes in this book have specific measurements for salt and pepper for a reason: Your mouth is more accurate than a measuring spoon. Taste and adjust as early and often as possible. (Oh, and get rid of that salt shaker! Put kosher salt in a small bowl by the stove and season with your fingers, which gives you real control and accuracy.)

2. When you salt is as important as how much you salt.

Season chicken, pork, and turkey up to 8 hours before cooking. The salt will penetrate the meat fully and yield juicier, more fully seasoned results. (That said, only season burgers seconds before throwing them onto the grill—otherwise the salt will break down the protein strands and create tougher patties.)

3. Fix your mistakes.

Too much salt? Use a splash of vinegar to provide a counterbalancing punch of acid. Too much heat? Try a drizzle of honey to mellow out the spice.

4. Shop for food on Monday or Tuesday before 10 a.m. or after 7 p.m.

Research shows that these are the least-crowded moments of the week at the market, making it the best time to pick out first-rate products without the clamoring masses.

5. Pat meat and fish dry before cooking.

Surface moisture creates steam when it hits a hot pan or grill, impeding caramelization. If your fish has skin, use a sharp knife to squeegee off the water trapped within it.

6. For deeply flavored foods, don't overcrowd the pan.

Ingredient overload makes a pan's temperature plummet, and foods end up steaming rather than caramelizing. This adds cooking time and subtracts flavor. All ingredients should fit comfortably in one layer, so use a pan that's big enough for the job, and cook in batches if necessary.

7. Don't scorch the nonstick!

Teflon can deteriorate over high heat, so save your nonstick pans for gentler tasks like cooking omelets and fish.

8. Nothing beats crispy chicken skin.

Buy a whole chicken the day before you'll cook it, sprinkle on a teaspoon of kosher salt, and leave it uncovered in the fridge. The air and salt will draw out excess water. Just be sure to pat dry with paper towels before cooking.

9. Think of a broiler as an inverted grill,

a source of concentrated, quick-cooking heat. Chicken, pork chops, and steaks take about 10 minutes to broil; just be sure to flip them mid-way through the cooking process.

10. Instantly improve your next TV dinner:

After cooking, add fresh herbs, a squeeze of citrus, and a drizzle of olive oil to transform any frozen entree.

11. Keep tomatoes out of the fridge.

Same with peaches, potatoes, onions, bread, garlic, and coffee. Cold temperatures compromise the flavor and texture of these staples.

12. Warm food served on a cold plate is a rookie mistake.

Heat your dishes in a 150°F oven for 10 minutes before plating a meal. On the flip side, lightly chilled plates (use your freezer) boost the freshness of cold dishes like summer salads.

13. Adapt at will.

Ingredients aren't set in stone. Mushrooms can stand in for eggplant if that's what you have. Don't want to spend $3 on a bunch of celery just to use a single rib? Omit it. You like pork chops more than chicken breast? Switch it. Point is, if you understand the basic techniques and know what tastes good together, the possibility for creation in the kitchen is infinite.

14. Shop with the seasons.

Sure, sometimes you just need a tomato, but there are three great reasons to shop in season: It's cheaper, it tastes better, and it's better for you (and the planet).

15. Make friends.

Talk to butchers, produce suppliers, and fishmongers before buying. They can steer you to the best ingredients. Your supermarket doesn't have a butcher? Find a new place to shop.

16. Freshen up limp vegetables.

Drop your aging produce into ice water before cooking. Plants wilt due to water loss; ice water penetrates their cells to restore crispness.

17. Get more pucker for the price!

Zap lemons, limes, or oranges for 15 seconds in the microwave before squeezing them. The fruit will yield twice as much juice.

18. Go to farmers' markets early or late.

Early arrivals get the first pick of all the prettiest produce; latecomers can score last-second deals from vendors looking to unload their goods.

19. Flip your meat more than once.

Research shows that near-constant flipping of steak, chicken, chops, and burgers not only allows your food to cook faster, but also more evenly. Aim for one flip per minute.

20. Give it a rest.

If you slice into meat right after it finishes cooking, precious juices will escape. Wait 5 minutes before biting into burgers or grilled chicken, 7 minutes before cutting into steaks, and 15 minutes before carving a large roast.

CHAPTER 2

BREAKFAST

America's Worst BREAKFASTS

IHOP's Big Steak Omelette

1,150 calories
78 g fat
(27 g saturated, 0.5 g trans)
2,390 mg sodium
Price: $8.99

We consider omelets a recipe for morning glory: Protein-rich eggs offer the perfect base for nutritious stuffers like veggies and lean meats. But this breakfast blunder from IHOP is no omelet; it's a mass of steak and cheese with a few eggs thrown in to hold it all together. And as if assaulting your arteries with an aggregate of animal fat wasn't enough, IHOP also stuffs this egg envelope with fried potatoes and its signature splash of pancake batter. Unfortunately, the infamous pancake purveyor isn't alone with this omelet offense. With few exceptions, big chains' massive portions and high-fat fillers make the morning specialty a dish best served at home.

Eat This Instead!
Mile-High Omelet (page 50)
280 calories
19 g fat (7 g saturated)
740 mg sodium
Cost per serving: $1.84
Save! 870 calories and $7.15!

Smoothie King's The Hulk Strawberry (40 oz)

1,810 calories
54 g fat (26 g saturated)
291g carbs
Price: $8.99

Disaster in a glass. Well, not so much a glass as a trough of terror, a 40-ounce nightmare of cheap fats and refined carbohydrates that Hollywood stars turn to when looking to put on weight for a new role. This isn't the only frightening smoothie out there—both Smoothie King and Jamba Juice are guilty of selling milk shakes disguised as health

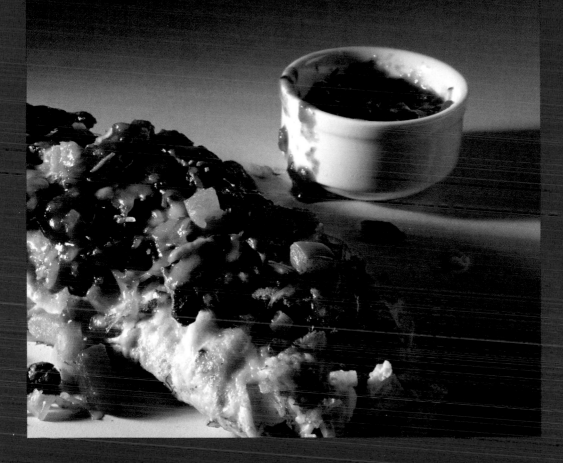

1,150 calories
IHOP's Big Steak Omelette: a rude awakening.

food. It's just the most potent reminder that a blender and a bag of frozen fruit can mean big savings in the wallet and even more in the waistline.

Eat This Instead!
Banana-Mango Smoothie
(page 44)

300 calories
2 g fat (1 g saturated)
70 g carbs
Cost per serving: $2.25
Save! 1,510 calories and $6.74!

WORST EGGS
Cheesecake Factory's Huevos Rancheros

1,100 calories
N/A g fat (27 g saturated)
1,470 mg sodium
Price: $9.95

English translation: country-style eggs. Cheesecake Factory translation: death by quesadillas. None of the chain's dietary transgressions shock us at this point, but it takes major cojones to take one of Mexico's most nutritious exports and turn it into a morning starter with more calories than half a dozen Taco Bell crunchy tacos. And how does the Factory pull off such a catastrophic calorie load? By replacing the dish's traditional corn tortillas with cheese-crammed quesadillas, topping it off with globs of sour cream, and serving it up in a portion more fit for a last meal than a first meal. *Dios mio!*

Eat This Instead!
Huevos Rancheros
(page 46)

480 calories
15 g fat (3 g saturated)
680 mg sodium
Cost per serving: $1.77
Save! 680 calories and $8.18!

WORST PANCAKES
IHOP's Strawberry Banana Pancakes
(4 pancakes with butter and strawberry syrup)

900 calories
32 g fat
(13 g saturated, 1.5 g trans)
71 g sugars
2,600 mg sodium
Price: $6.99

Pancakes. The name says it all: they're dessert disguised as breakfast. But there's good news: There are ways to satisfy your a.m. sweet tooth without foiling your get-fit plans. These plate-sized banana behemoths from IHOP just ain't one of 'em. Besides the fruit, there's just nothing nutritionally redeeming about these pitiful pancakes. All you have here is a boatload of empty carbs, a flood of syrupy strawberry sauce, a whipping of whipped cream, and, most astoundingly, more than one and a half days' worth of sodium. A pancake is only as good as its ingredients, and ours are made with ricotta cheese, a bit of whole-wheat flour, and thick slices of fresh banana.

Eat This Instead!
Banana Pancakes
(page 48)

320 calories
5 g fat
(1.5 g saturated)
320 mg sodium
Cost per serving: $1.49
Save! 580 calories and $5.50!

WORST BREAKFAST
Cheesecake Factory's Bruleed French Toast

2,560 calories
N/A g fat
(89 g saturated fat)
198 g carbs
Price: $11.95

True to its namesake, this sorry breakfast plate attempts to make up for its nutritional shortcomings by enticing diners with indulgent ingredients like cream-drenched bread, piles of pecans, and a snowstorm of powdered sugar. But behind all that overcompensation is a morning meal—otherwise known as the single worst breakfast in America—with more calories than three slices of the chain's Fresh Strawberry Cheesecake.

Eat This Instead!
Vanilla-Bourbon French Toast (page 52)

330 calories
8 g fat (3 g saturated)
44 g carbs
Cost per serving: $1.40
Save! 2,2300 calories and $10.55!

2,910 calories

The French Toast Napoleon from the Cheesecake Factory is the single worst meal in America.

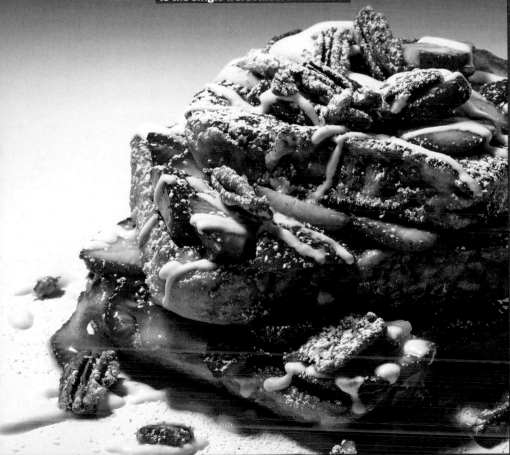

The Breakfast Sandwich

Eggs have gotten a bad rap. No, the Egg Advisory Board hasn't put the screws on us; we just call it like we see it. Reams of research in recent years have shown that moderate consumption of eggs has no negative effect on cholesterol, and some studies have gone as far as arguing that egg consumption can actually boost good cholesterol. All of this is to confirm what we've been saying for years: There are few better ways to start your day than with an egg or two.

Four Handheld Heroes

The vessel and the toppings may change, but one thing remains constant: These savory breakfast sandwiches are a perfect start to your day.

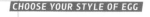

CHOOSE YOUR STYLE OF EGG

To minimize calories, use a nonstick pan or cast-iron skillet coated with a few drops of olive oil.

FRIED

CHOOSE YOUR PROTEIN

Want perfect bacon every time? Bake in a 375°F oven for 15 minutes.

BACON

HAM

TURKEY

CHOOSE YOUR PRODUCE

Fresh baby spinach or wilted spinach are both excellent with fried or scrambled eggs.

SPINACH

AVOCADO

CHOOSE YOUR ADD-ONS

Bottled is fine, or try our Pico de Gallo on page 319.

SALSA

GUACAMOLE

SRIRACHA/HOT SAUCE

CHOOSE YOUR VESSEL

CORN TORTILLAS

WHOLE-WHEAT WRAP

TACO
Scrambled eggs + bacon + spinach + salsa + corn tortilla

WRAP
Scrambled eggs + chicken sausage + diced tomato + guacamole + whole-wheat wrap

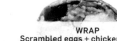

Matrix

SCRAMBLED

Don't be scared! Bring 6 inches of water (plus a tablespoon of white vinegar) to a simmer. Crack the egg into a glass then slip it gently into the water. Cook until the white fully sets, about 2 minutes.

POACHED

Regular pork sausage has no place on the breakfast menu (or any menu, for that matter). Chicken sausage is every bit as delicious for half the calories.

CHICKEN SAUSAGE

CANADIAN BACON

Packs about one-quarter the fat of regular pork bacon.

TOMATO

ARUGULA

ROASTED PEPPERS

American or Swiss are your lightest options for sliced cheese. Otherwise, try a pinch of shredded cheese to keep the calories down.

CHEESE

Try mixing thick, creamy yogurt with hot sauce or pesto for a perfect breakfast condiment.

GREEK YOGURT

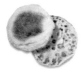

ENGLISH MUFFIN

WHOLE-GRAIN BREAD

PITA

MUFFIN
Poached egg + Canadian bacon + avocado
+ roasted peppers + hot sauce + English muffin

SANDWICH
Fried egg + ham + arugula + tomato
+ sriracha + yogurt + whole-grain bread

The Rules of the Breakfast Sandwich

Master the egg
The egg is the star and it deserves a bit of attention. If scrambling, use low heat and a constant stirring motion to create soft curds. If frying, cook the egg in olive oil over a steady medium flame just until the white sets.

Make it moist
Nobody wants a dry sandwich, and the same holds true in the morning hours. Salsa and hot sauce are the most obvious additions, but guacamole, pesto, chimichurri, and garlic- and herb-spiked yogurt all make incredible additions to the final package.

Pack on the produce
Most people think of breakfast sandwiches as meat-and-cheese affairs, but you should view them as the perfect opportunity to sneak some vegetation into your diet. Arugula adds a spicy kick, roasted peppers bring smoky sweetness, and avocado contributes fiber, healthy fat, and incredible richness to the table.

Banana-Mango Smoothie

There's something deeply rewarding about starting your day with a great smoothie. Not just because you know you're doing your body a favor, but also because a well-made smoothie tastes like it should be bad for you— at turns sweet and smooth, creamy and tart. Know what's especially comforting about this recipe? It doesn't come loaded with added sugars and it doesn't cost $7. Rejoice.

You'll Need:

- 1 ripe banana
- ¾ cup frozen mango pieces
- ½ cup orange juice
- ¼ cup Greek yogurt

How to Make It:

- Place all ingredients into a blender and blend until smooth and creamy, at least 30 seconds. If the smoothie is too thick (which depends on the size of the banana), add a few splashes of water and blend again.

Makes 1 serving

Per Serving
$2.25
300 calories
2 g fat
(1 g saturated)
70 g carbs

SECRET WEAPON

Frozen Fruit

Frozen fruit is often looked upon as a second-class citizen in the produce world, but it's the secret ingredient in a first-rate smoothie. Not only does frozen fruit give you a cold smoothie without the diluting effects of ice, it also lends a thick, creamy body to the final product. The nutritional advantages may be even greater. Studies have found that many nutrients are higher in frozen fruits and vegetables than in fresh, since frozen fruits are picked at the height of their season and frozen immediately, while "fresh" fruits often take weeks before landing in your shopping cart.

3 More Power Smoothies

THE CAFFEINATED BANANA

- 1 very ripe banana
- ½ cup strong coffee
- ½ cup milk
- 1 Tbsp peanut butter
- 1 Tbsp agave syrup
- 1 cup ice

THE BLUE MONSTER

- 1 cup frozen blueberries
- ½ cup pomegranate or blueberry juice
- ½ cup yogurt
- 3 or 4 cubes of ice
- 1 Tbsp flaxseed

PAPAYA BERRY

- ¾ cup frozen papaya
- ¾ cup frozen strawberries
- ½ cup milk
- ½ cup orange juice
- 1 Tbsp fresh mint

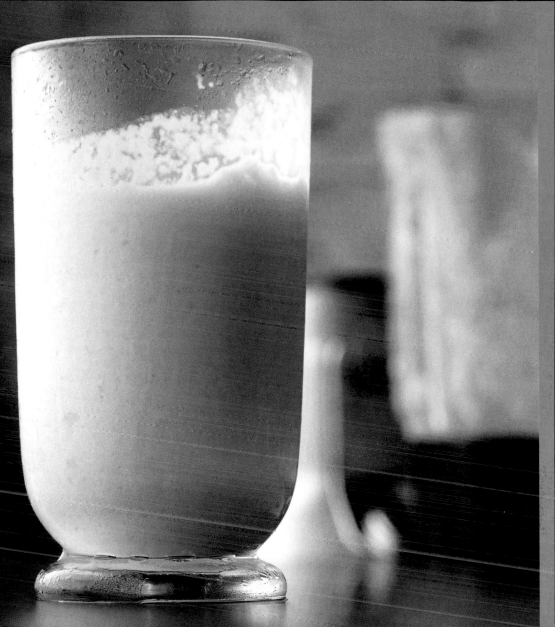

Huevos Rancheros

This is the type of breakfast you want when you really need to deliver on the day. Not only are huevos rancheros one of the most delicious morning creations of all time, their balance of protein, fiber, and antioxidants is designed to keep you at the top of your game all day long, too.

You'll Need:

1 can (16 oz) whole peeled tomatoes, with juice

½ small onion, chopped

1 clove garlic, chopped

1 Tbsp chopped chipotle pepper

¼ cup chopped fresh cilantro

Juice of 1 lime

Salt and black pepper to taste

1 can (16 oz) black beans

Pinch of ground cumin

8 eggs

8 corn tortillas

How to Make It:

- Combine the tomatoes, onion, garlic, chipotle, cilantro, and half of the lime juice in a food processor and pulse until well blended but still slightly chunky. Season with salt and pepper.

- Mix the black beans, cumin, and remaining lime juice in a bowl; season with salt and pepper. Use the back of a fork to lightly mash up the beans, adding a splash of warm water if necessary.

- Coat a large nonstick skillet or sauté pan with nonstick cooking spray and heat over medium heat. Break the eggs into the skillet; cook until the whites have set but the yolks are still loose and runny.

- On a separate burner, heat a medium skillet over medium heat and add the tortillas, 2 at a time; cook for 1 minute on each side, until lightly toasted.

- To assemble the dish, spread the tortillas with the beans, top with the eggs, and top the eggs with the salsa. Garnish with more cilantro, if you like, and serve immediately.

Makes 4 servings

Per Serving
$1.77
480 calories
15 g fat
(3 g saturated)
680 mg sodium

SECRET WEAPON

Chipotle pepper

We admit to having an overwhelming infatuation with these canned chiles, but once you recognize their potential for adding instant flavor to a dish, you will, too. Chipotles are smoked jalapeños, and they come canned with a spicy, vinegary tomato sauce called adobo. You'll see a lot of recipes in this book that call for chipotles, so here's what you do: Buy a can, dump the whole thing into a blender or food processor, and pulse. Use a spoonful to spike salsas, marinades, mashed potatoes, and soups. Beyond being insanely delicious, the capsaicin in chipotle has been shown to boost metabolism.

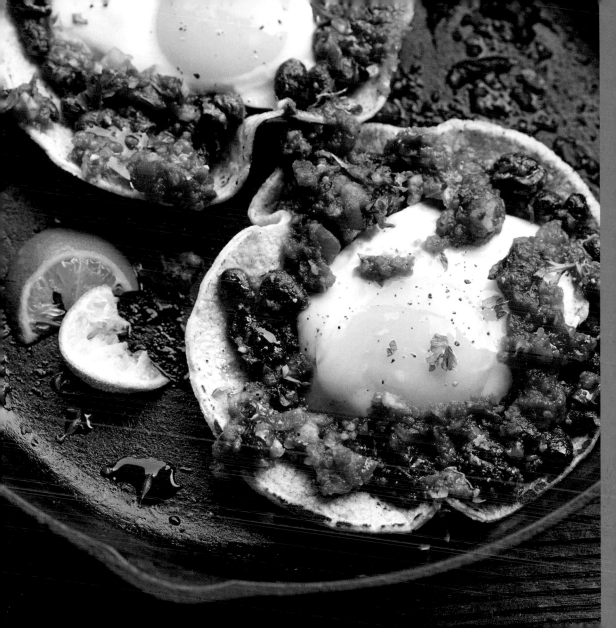

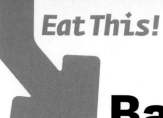

Banana Pancakes

Using yogurt and cottage cheese in these pancakes does two things: It brings extra protein to the breakfast table, and it helps produce the lightest, moistest pancakes you've ever tasted. The addition of fresh slices of banana, which caramelize into golden-brown disks of sweetness once they hit the skillet, to the batter can never be a bad thing, but the secret here is in the batter recipe, which should become your go-to base for all pancakes moving forward.

You'll Need:

- 1 **cup plain 2% Greek yogurt**
- 1 **cup low-fat cottage cheese or ricotta cheese**
- 3 **eggs**

Juice of 1 lemon

- 1 **cup white whole wheat flour (we like King Arthur's)**
- ½ **tsp baking soda**

Pinch of salt

- 2 **bananas, sliced**

Warm maple syrup for serving

How to Make It:

- Whisk together the yogurt, cottage cheese, eggs, and lemon juice in a bowl. Mix the flour, baking soda, and salt in another bowl. Add the flour mixture to the yogurt mixture and stir just until blended.

- Heat a large skillet or sauté pan over medium-low heat. Coat with nonstick cooking spray and add batter in large spoonfuls (about 2 tablespoons each). As soon as the batter hits the pan, add three or four banana slices directly to each pancake, gently pressing them into the batter. Cook for 3 to 5 minutes, until the tops begin to bubble. Flip the pancakes and cook on the second sides for 3 minutes longer, until browned.

- It will take a few batches to get through the batter, depending on the size of your skillet. You can keep the pancakes warm in a 200°F oven while you work through the batches. Serve with more sliced bananas and a drizzle of syrup.

Makes 4 servings

Per Serving
$1.49
320 calories
5 g fat
(1.5 g saturated)
54 g carbs

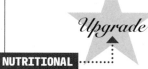

Upgrade

NUTRITIONAL

Most supermarket syrups are junk, made almost entirely of high-fructose corn syrup and chemical additives designed to approximate a maple flavor. But real maple syrup can be prohibitively expensive. Solution? Fruit compote. Take a bag of frozen fruit (blueberries, strawberries, mixed berries), dump into a saucepan with ½ cup water and ¼ cup sugar, and simmer for 10 minutes, until the fruit is warm and the mixture has thickened. Use it for all your pancake and waffle needs.

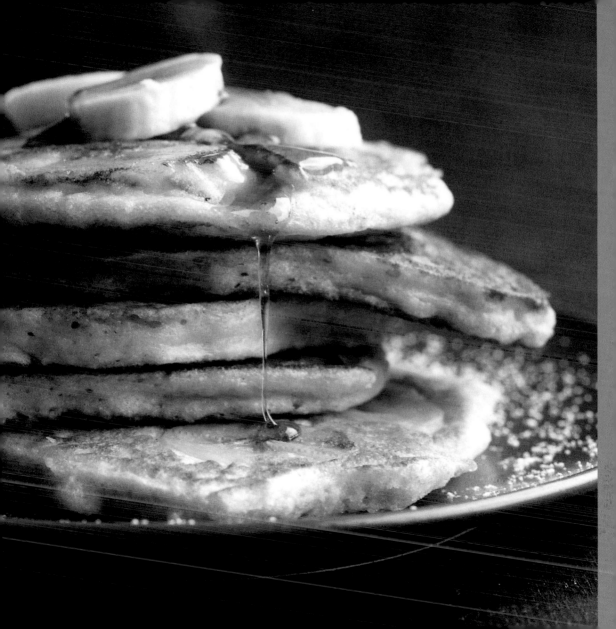

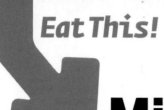

Mile-High Omelets

The classic diner omelet is an oversize envelope of eggs soaked in cheap oil and bulging with fatty fillers. The damage, with toast and hash browns: about 1,400 calories and 70 grams of fat. Our ode to Denver doesn't cut the cheese or the meat or even turn to Egg Beaters. No, this is just honest cooking with good ingredients in reasonable portions, exactly what an omelet should be.

You'll Need:

- ½ Tbsp olive oil, plus more for cooking the omelets
- 1 green bell pepper, diced
- 4 oz cremini or button mushrooms, sliced
- 1 small onion, diced
- 4 oz smoked ham, cubed or sliced into thin strips
- Salt and black pepper to taste
- 8 eggs
- 2 Tbsp 2% milk
- ½ cup shredded sharp Cheddar

How to Make It:

- Heat the olive oil in a medium sauté pan over medium heat. Add the bell pepper, mushrooms, and onions and cook for about 7 minutes, until the vegetables are soft and lightly browned. Add the ham, cook for 1 minute more, then season with salt and pepper.

- Combine the eggs and milk and whisk until fully blended. Season with a few pinches of salt.

- Heat a small nonstick pan over medium heat. Swirl with just enough olive oil to coat. Ladle in one-quarter of the eggs and as soon as they begin to set, use a wooden spoon to scrape the egg from the bottom, working from one side of the pan to the other (like you were scrambling eggs). Stop scraping just before the egg is fully cooked, then spread one-quarter of the cheese and one-quarter of the vegetable mixture across the omelet. Use a spatula to carefully fold the egg over on itself. Slide the omelet out onto a warm plate. Repeat to make 4 omelets.

Makes 4 servings

Per Serving
$1.84
280 calories
19 g fat
(7 g saturated)
740 mg sodium

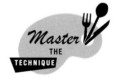

Master **THE** **TECHNIQUE**

Super-Fluffy Omelets

Achieve a soufflé-like texture with any omelet with one simple move. Combine the eggs and a splash of milk in a blender as you heat up your pan. Blend for 20 seconds, then add the eggs directly to the pan. The action from the blender helps whip air into the eggs, creating a tender curd and pillowy texture as the eggs cook.

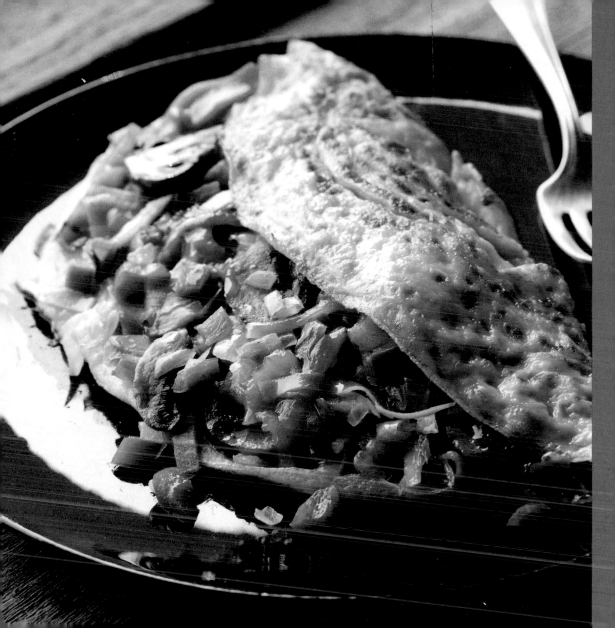

Eat This!

Vanilla-Bourbon French Toast

In France, French toast is called *pain perdu*—"lost bread," a nod to the fact that the dish works best with stale bread. More importantly, pain perdu isn't served at breakfast, but rather as a dessert, a reminder that this dish is traditionally soaked in sugar and cream. This version forgoes cream for milk, and a deluge of sugar for vanilla and a slug of bourbon. It's still a pretty decadent way to start your day, but at least you won't need a nap afterward.

You'll Need:

- 4 eggs
- 1½ cups 2% milk
- ¼ cup bourbon
- 1 tsp vanilla extract
- 1 Tbsp sugar
- ¼ tsp ground nutmeg
- 1 loaf day-old country bread, preferably whole wheat, cut into 8 slices

Butter for the pan

Maple or agave syrup for serving

How to Make It:

- Preheat the oven to 225°F.
- Combine the eggs, milk, bourbon, vanilla, sugar, and nutmeg in a shallow baking dish and whisk to combine. Soak each slice of bread for 30 seconds, turning once, before cooking.
- Heat a large cast-iron skillet or nonstick pan over medium heat. Melt a small pat of butter in the pan, enough to coat the surface. Add 2 to 4 slices of the soaked bread and cook for about 3 minutes, until a deep brown crust forms. Flip the bread and continue cooking for another 2 to 3 minutes, until golden brown and firm to the touch. Keep the cooked French toast in the oven while you work through the rest of the batch.
- Serve with warm syrup and a dusting of powdered sugar, if you like.

Makes 4 servings

Per Serving
$1.40
330 calories
8 g fat
(3 g saturated)
44 g carbs

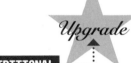

Upgrade

NUTRITIONAL

While we've managed to take most of the sting out of the French toast, it's still by definition a carb-heavy breakfast. But by increasing your fiber intake, you can blunt the impact on your blood sugar levels. Try replacing the syrup with any of the following:

- Sliced bananas, either raw or caramelized in a pan over medium heat for a few minutes
- Raw strawberries with powdered sugar
- Blueberries cooked for 15 minutes with a spoonful of water and sugar

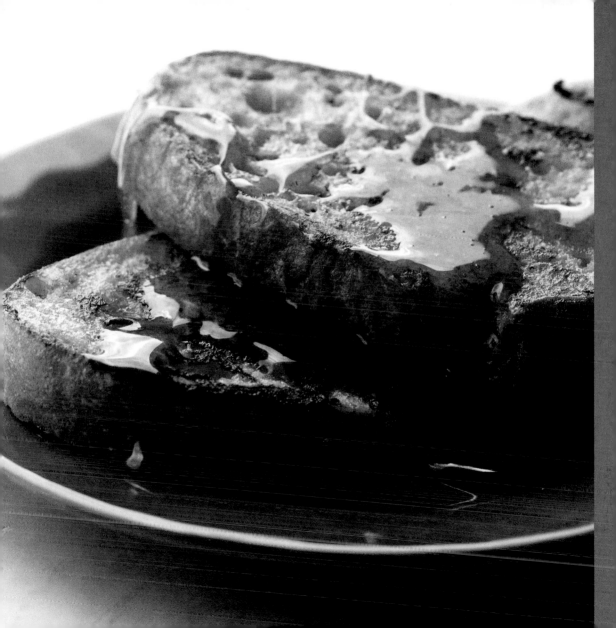

Shiitake, Spinach & Goat Cheese Scramble

Skillfully scrambled eggs are a joy on their own, but by taking the next step and folding in a few supporting players, you accomplish two goals: First, you make a simple breakfast suddenly taste and feel like something special. But also, most additions you can introduce to a sauté pan will further boost the nutritional profile of the heroic egg. For soft, extra-creamy scrambled eggs, make sure to turn the heat down and stir the eggs constantly.

You'll Need:

- 1½ Tbsp butter
- 1 cup sliced shiitake mushrooms
- 1 cup frozen spinach, thawed
- Salt and black pepper to taste
- 8 eggs
- 2 Tbsp 2% milk
- ½ cup fresh goat cheese

Per Serving
$1.98
240 calories
17 g fat
(5 g saturated)
640 mg sodium

How to Make It:

- Heat 1 tablespoon of the butter in a large nonstick pan over medium heat. When bubbling, add the shiitakes and cook for about 5 minutes, until lightly browned. Remove and reserve on a plate.

- In the same pan, sauté the spinach until heated all the way through. Season with salt and pepper. Transfer to a colander and squeeze out any excess water.

- Combine the eggs and the milk in a large bowl. Season with salt and whisk thoroughly. Add the remaining ½ tablespoon butter to the pan, turn the heat to low, and add the eggs. Use a wooden spoon to stir the eggs constantly, scraping the bottom of the pan to create small, delicate curds. Continue stirring in this manner for about 5 minutes, until the eggs are still very soft and loose. Add the mushrooms, spinach, and goat cheese and cook for about 2 minutes longer. Season to taste with black pepper.

Makes 4 servings

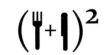

$$(\Upsilon + |)^2$$

MEAL MULTIPLIER

Other ways to bolster a breakfast scramble:

- Asparagus, feta, and cherry tomatoes
- Baby shrimp, garlic, and scallions
- Chicken sausage, mushrooms, scallions, and sharp Cheddar

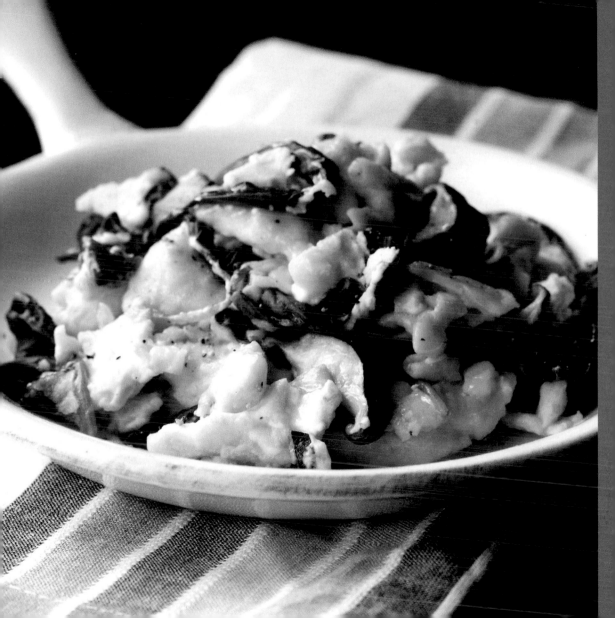

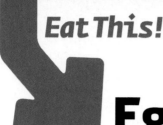

Eggs in Purgatory

It was a long night, and you feel every last drop of it when your feet hit the floor the next morning. Your head is pounding, your stomach is stirring, your body needs nourishment. Not a pile of greasy potatoes, but real food: protein, good carbs, a bit of healthy fat. But not just nutrients—flavors, too: spicy, sweet, creamy, salty. That's where these eggs come into play. They offer layers of intense flavors built around some of the healthiest ingredients in the pantry (tomatoes, garlic, whole grains). We like to call this our Hangover Helper.

You'll Need:

- ½ cup farro or barley
- ½ Tbsp olive oil
- 2 oz pancetta or bacon, diced
- ½ medium onion, diced
- 2 cloves garlic, minced
- ½ tsp red pepper flakes
- 1 can (28 oz) crushed tomatoes

Salt and black pepper to taste

- 8 eggs

Farro, an Italian grain loaded with fiber, also goes by the name emmer. Barley or even brown rice make fine substitutes.

How to Make It:

- Bring a pot of water to a boil over high heat. Add the farro or barley and cook for about 20 minutes, until just tender. Drain.

- While the grains cook, heat the olive oil in the largest cast-iron skillet or sauté pan you have. Cook the pancetta until lightly browned, then add the onion, garlic, and red pepper flakes and cook for about 3 minutes, until the onions are softened. Stir in the tomatoes and the farro or barley and simmer for 5 minutes, until slightly reduced. Season with salt and black pepper.

- Use the back of a large serving spoon to make 8 small wells in the sauce. Crack an egg into each well. Cook over low heat for about 7 minutes, until the whites set but the yolks are still runny. You can use your fork to break up the whites so they cook more quickly.

- Serve with whole-wheat toast for scooping up the sauce.

Makes 4 servings

Per Serving
$1.68
360 calories
17 g fat
(5 g saturated)
680 mg sodium

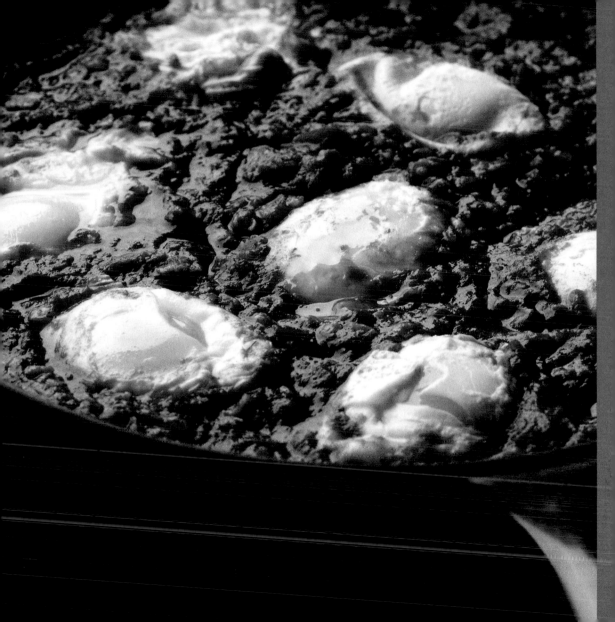

Eat This!

Spinach & Ham Quiche

The quiche is the ultimate culinary chameleon, not just because it can be made with dozens of different flavor combinations, but also because it's as good for breakfast with a cup of coffee as it is for dinner with a glass of red wine. Or split the difference: Make this for Sunday night's dinner and then take a wedge with you to work on Monday; it makes for a fine desk-side lunch.

You'll Need:

- 1 frozen pie shell, thawed and pricked with a fork
- ½ Tbsp olive oil
- 1 clove garlic, minced
- ½ bunch spinach, washed, dried, and stemmed
- 2 oz smoked ham, cut into ¼-inch cubes
- ½ cup shredded Swiss cheese, such as Gruyère
- 4 eggs
- ¾ cup milk
- ¼ cup half-and-half
- ½ tsp salt
- Pinch of nutmeg

How to Make It:

- Preheat the oven to 375°F. When hot, place the pie shell on the middle rack and bake for about 8 minutes, until lightly toasted, but not browned.

- While the oven heats and the shell bakes, heat the olive oil in large skillet or pot over medium heat. Add the garlic, cook for 30 seconds, then add the spinach. Cook for 5 minutes, until the spinach is fully wilted. In a large mixing bowl, combine the ham, cheese, eggs, milk, half-and-half, and spinach, squeezing the spinach thoroughly before adding to purge any excess water. Season with salt and a pinch of nutmeg.

- Pour the egg mixture into the warm pastry shell. Bake for about 12 minutes, until the quiche has browned lightly on top and a toothpick inserted into the center comes out clean.

Makes 6 servings

Per Serving
$1.21
260 calories
15 g fat
(6 g saturated)
550 mg sodium

$(\dagger + \textbf{I})^2$

MEAL MULTIPLIER

Other winning quiche combinations:

- Artichoke hearts, sun-dried tomatoes, feta cheese
- Shredded rotisserie chicken, sautéed mushrooms, and asparagus
- Diced Spanish chorizo, roasted red pepper, ricotta cheese

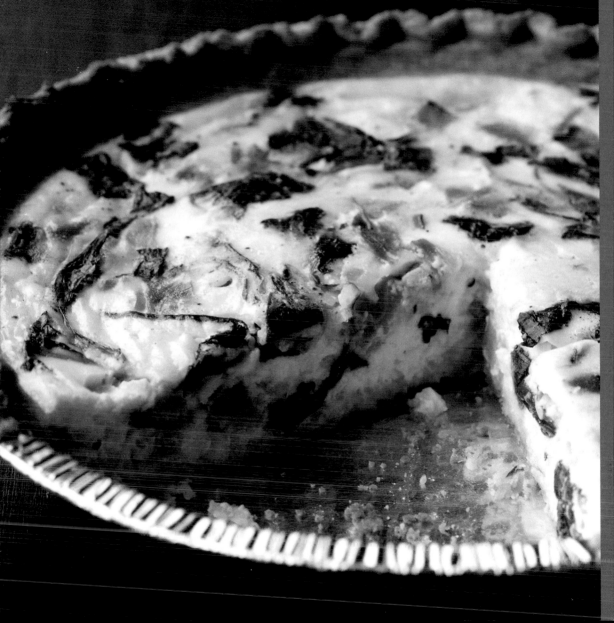

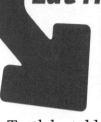

Eat This!

Flaky Southern Biscuits

Truth be told, a low-calorie biscuit is no easy feat. You can make one with yogurt or some funky butter substitute instead of the real thing, but you'll know something is amiss the second you bite down. Where's the flakiness? Where's the comfort? To keep the biscuit as healthy as possible while still producing a genuine, flaky, Southern-style treasure, we've cut out the shortening (trans fats are so 1990s), showed some restraint with the butter, and used low-fat buttermilk to bring moisture and tang to the mix.

You'll Need:

- 2 cups all-purpose flour
- 4 Tbsp cold butter
- 4 tsp baking powder
- ¼ tsp baking soda
- ½ tsp salt
- 1 cup low-fat buttermilk

How to Make It:

- Preheat the oven to 425°F.
- Combine the flour, butter, baking powder, baking soda, and salt in large mixing bowl. Use your fingers to break up the butter, mashing it into the flour to create little pebbles. When the flour and butter have been combined, make a well in the center of the mixture and pour in the buttermilk. Use a fork to gently bring the dough together.
- Dump the dough out onto a floured surface and pat it out into a square. Gently fold the dough onto itself four or five times (this action helps create tall, delicate biscuits), then roll it out to form a 1"-thick circle. Use a round cookie cutter (or even a drinking glass) to cut out the biscuits. (You should get about 6 from the original circle.) Re-form another circle and repeat. You should have about 10 biscuits in total.
- Arrange the biscuits on a baking sheet coated with nonstick spray. Bake on the middle rack for 10 to 12 minutes, until golden brown.

Makes 10 biscuits

Per Serving
$0.19
140 calories
5 g fat
(3 g saturated)
370 mg sodium

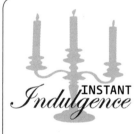

Instant **INSTANT** *Indulgence*

These biscuits are perfect on their own, but we never shy away from gilding the lily a bit. A few biscuit fillers to get you started:

- Scrambled egg with scallion and sharp Cheddar, topped with salsa
- Orange marmalade and smoked ham
- Grilled chicken drizzled with honey and hot sauce

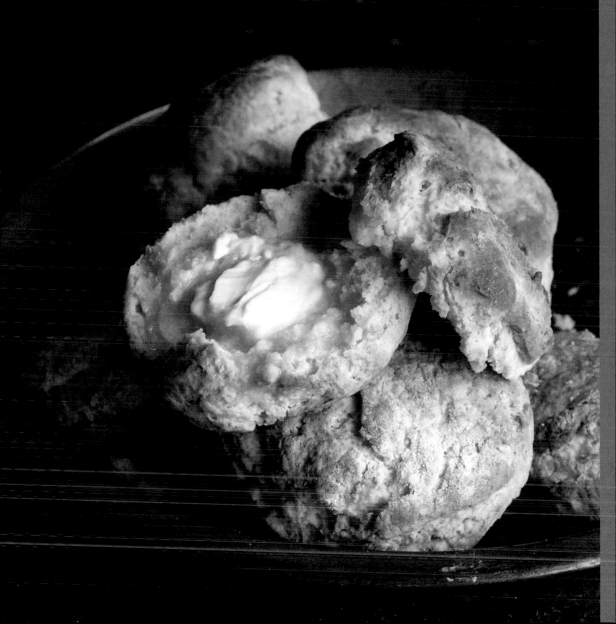

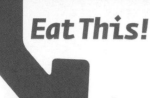

Steak & Eggs with Chimichurri

There's nothing subtle about the commingling of seared steak and egg yolk in the morning. You know you're in for something serious even before it hits the table. Amazingly enough, though, this is a near-perfect nutritional start to your day, loaded with protein, healthy fat, and even a bit of fiber. This meal works as well at 11:30 a.m., as a cure for a hangover or post-workout hunger pangs, as it does at 8 p.m., as a remedy for a long day at work.

You'll Need:

- 1 Tbsp olive oil
- 1 lb flank or skirt steak
- Salt and black pepper to taste
- 4 Roma tomatoes, halved lengthwise
- 4 eggs
- Chimichurri (page 319)

How to Make It:

- Heat ½ tablespoon of the olive oil in a grill pan or cast-iron skillet over high heat. Season the steak all over with salt and pepper. Cook, turning the steak every minute or so, for 7 to 8 minutes total, until fully browned on the outside and firm but fully yielding to the touch. Remove to a cutting board and rest for 5 minutes before slicing.

- While the steak rests, place the tomatoes cut-side down in the same pan and cook for about 2 minutes, until the bottoms are lightly blackened.

- Heat the remaining ½ tablespoon olive oil in a large nonstick pan. Working in batches, crack the eggs into the pan and fry until sunny-side up, the whites just set and the yolks still loose. Season with salt and black pepper.

- Slice the steak against the natural grain of the meat. Divide among 4 warm plates with the eggs and tomatoes. Spoon chimichurri liberally over the steak and eggs.

Makes 4 servings

Per Serving
$3.30
400 calories
23 g fat
(5 g saturated)
660 mg sodium

SECRET WEAPON

Chimichurri

This bright green garlic and parsley sauce is Argentina's most ubiquitous condiment for a reason: It has that unique power to make almost everything taste better. Grilled steak and chimi is the classic combo, but it makes even more sense when you add eggs to the picture. Beyond beef, try chimichurri as a sandwich spread, as a topping for roast chicken or grilled fish, or as a dipping sauce for grilled asparagus or crispy roasted potatoes. It keeps for a week in the fridge and gets better with time, so make up a big batch and go to town.

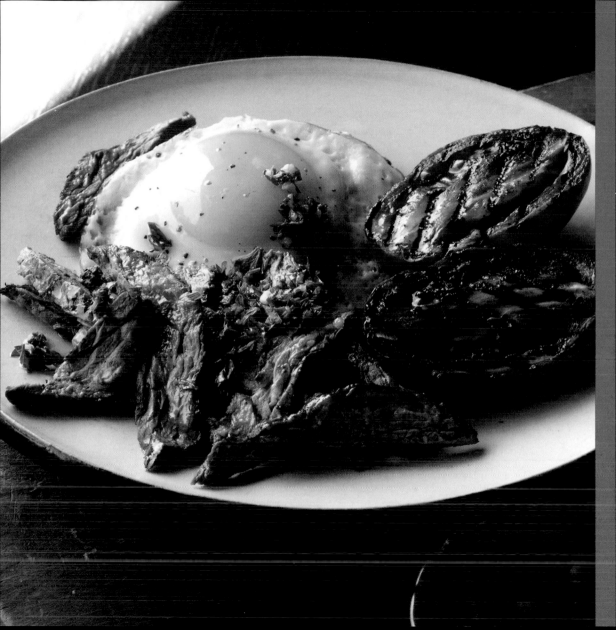

CHAPTER 3

APPETIZERS

America's Worst APPETIZERS

Uno Chicago Grill's Buffalo Wings

1,340 calories
108 g fat (25 g saturated)
3,530 mg sodium
Price: $9.99

Surprisingly, wings are often one of the best apps on any chain menu—they're comprised primarily of protein, and while they've usually taken a dip in hot oil, their slight stature minimizes the deep-fried damage. Not so surprising? Uno Chicago's version is the worst we've seen. The chain has a propensity for greasy grub, so we're guessing the colossal calorie count of this chicken plate comes from an unnecessarily oily buffalo sauce. Either way, a few (unbreaded) wings are usually a safe bet at your favorite chain, and an even smarter choice at home, where you can roast them in the oven or crisp them up on the grill.

Eat This Instead!
Roasted Wings with Blue Cheese Yogurt (page 70)
300 calories
23 g fat (7 g saturated)
540 mg sodium
Cost per serving: $1.31
Save! 1,040 calories and $8.68!

Applebee's Spinach and Artichoke Dip

1,570 calories
105 g fat
(27 g saturated, 1 g trans)
2,720 mg sodium
Price: $7.99

Spinach: excellent. Artichoke: fantastic. Any restaurant dip combining the two: nutritional mayhem. To be fair, most chip dips are inherently corrupt. More often than not, their creamy texture depends on high-fat ingredients like cheese, sour cream, and mayo, and their semi-liquid state makes it easy to scoop up half

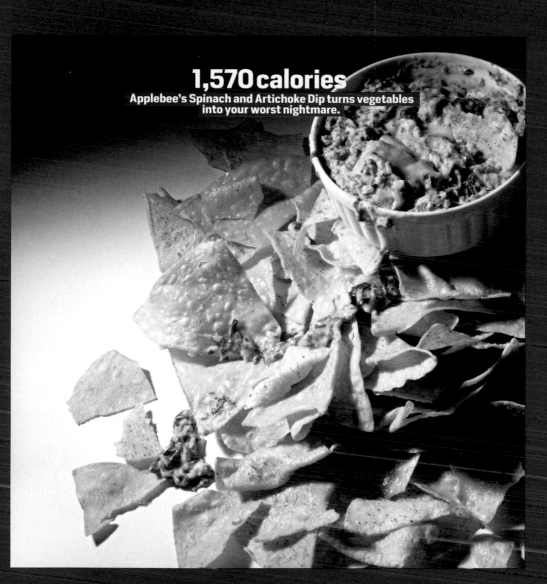

1,570 calories

Applebee's Spinach and Artichoke Dip turns vegetables into your worst nightmare.

a day's calories without even realizing it. Add that to the fact that most chain dips are accompanied by a heap of deep-fried tortilla chips (we're looking at you, Applebee's), and it's no surprise that this healthy-sounding starter will finish off your diet in one fell scoop.

Eat This Instead!
Spinach-Artichoke Dip
(page 74)

270 calories
10 g fat (2.5 g saturated)
520 mg sodium
Cost per serving: $2.07
Save! 1,300 calories and $5.92!

Ruby Tuesday's Baja Chicken Quesadilla

1,604 calories
104 g fat
(N/A g saturated)
4,744 mg sodium
Price: $7.99

Quesadillas rival nachos as the most treacherous Mexican-inspired offerings on America's big-chain menus. Prodigious portions and greasy tortillas certainly don't help matters, but the real perpetrator of the quesadilla's undoing is the cheese. It takes a ton of queso to glue together otherwise-healthy fillers like veggies and lean meat, which results in disasters like this Tuesday's offering, which derives nearly 60 percent of its calories from fat.

Eat This Instead!
Crispy Quesadillas
(page 84)

310 calories
16 g fat
(5 g saturated)
730 mg sodium
Cost per serving: $3.11
Save! 1,294 calories and $6.88!

Cheesecake Factory's Nachos with Spicy Chicken

1,930 calories
N/A g fat
(61 g saturated)
2,944 mg sodium
Price: $11.95

Truth be told, we've never come across a plate of restaurant nachos worth the caloric investment, and this Factory option is the worst in the land. We get that this plate is meant for sharing, but even if you split it with three friends, you're still taking in a meal's worth of calories before your entrée hits the table. The bottom line: An appetizer should stimulate your appetite, not suffocate it with enough cheese and sour scream to feed a small Mexican village.

Eat This Instead!
Nachos with Chicken and Black Beans (page 72)

330 calories
12 g fat (6 g saturated)
500 mg sodium
Cost per serving: $2.65
Save! 1,600 calories and $9.30!

Chili's Texas Cheese Fries with Chili and Ranch

2,150 calories
144 g fat (62 g saturated)
6,080 mg sodium
Price: $8.29

Everything is bigger in Texas, they like to say, including calorie counts and fat content. Essentially a plate of nachos that replaces chips with fries, this appetizer is far and away the most offensive on the Chili's menu, and one of the worst in the country. It dishes out the caloric equivalent of 22 of the chain's deep-fried mozzarella sticks, and a sodium count that will give your blood-pressure reading the Lone-Star treatment to boot.

Eat This Instead!
Cheese Fries (page 78)

300 calories
13 g fat (5 g saturated)
310 mg sodium
Cost per serving: $1.21
Save! 1,850 calories and $7.08!

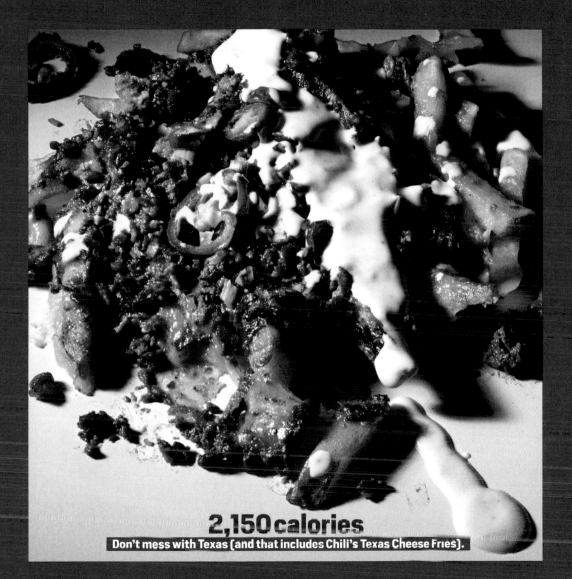

2,150 calories
Don't mess with Texas (and that includes Chili's Texas Cheese Fries).

Roasted Wings with Blue Cheese Yogurt

The deep fryer adds two very important things to chicken wings: crunch and calories. We will happily take the former, but not at the steep cost of the latter. Instead, we turn to a trick we first discovered from SeriousEats.com writer J. Kenji López-Alt, who found that the addition of baking powder and salt hours before cooking helps extract unwanted moisture from chicken skin, paving the way for a crispy oven-baked wing—the best of both worlds.

You'll Need:

- 2 lb chicken wings
- 1 tsp baking powder
- 1 tsp kosher salt
- 2 Tbsp butter
- 2 Tbsp Frank's RedHot pepper sauce

Juice of 1 lemon

- ½ cup Greek yogurt
- 1 clove garlic, finely minced
- 2 Tbsp crumbled blue cheese

How to Make It:

- Toss the wings with the baking powder and salt and spread out on a large baking sheet. Refrigerate, uncovered, for at least 2 hours, or up to 8 hours. (If pressed for time, this step can be skipped entirely.)
- Preheat the oven to 425°F. Roast the wings for about 35 minutes, until nicely browned and crisp.
- While the wings roast, combine the butter, hot sauce, and half of the lemon juice in a large sauté pan set over medium heat. Cook until the butter has fully melted and incorporated with the hot sauce to create a uniform sauce.
- In a medium bowl, combine the yogurt, garlic, and remaining lemon juice. Stir in the blue cheese.
- Place the wings in a large bowl and pour the hot sauce over the top. Toss to thoroughly coat. Serve with the blue cheese yogurt.

Makes 6 to 8 servings

Per Serving
$1.31
300 calories
23 g fat
(7 g saturated)
540 mg sodium

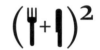

$(\Psi + \mathbf{I})^2$

MEAL MULTIPLIER

The global pantry holds the keys to opening new worlds of wing potential. Follow the same roasting technique for the wings, then toss them with any of the following combos just before serving:

- 2 tablespoons butter, 2 tablespoons honey, 1 tablespoon chipotle pepper, juice of 1 lime
- 2 tablespoons butter, 2 tablespoons soy sauce, 1 tablespoon sriracha, juice of 1 lime
- ¼ cup coconut milk, 1 tablespoon red curry powder, juice of 1 lime

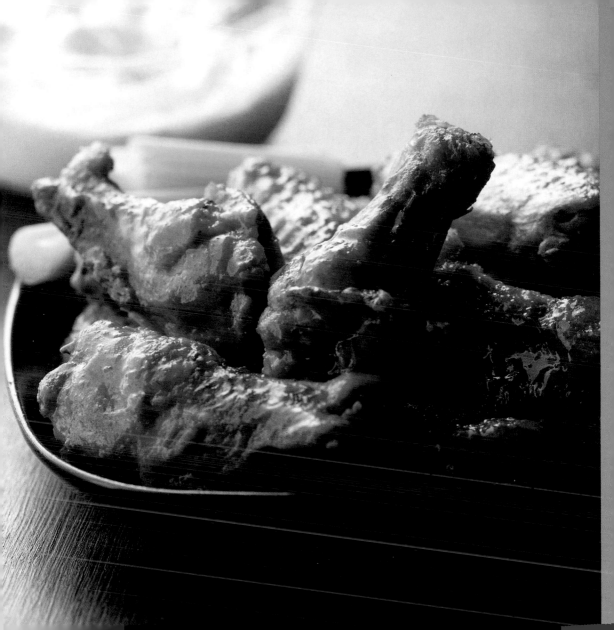

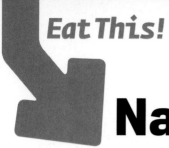

Eat This!

Nachos with Chicken & Black Beans

We've never found a nacho worth recommending in the restaurant world. The sad truth is that the tortilla chips are rendered helpless vessels for thousands of calories of cheese, sour cream, and oily ground beef. And besides, who wants to dig through soggy nacho detritus in search of a chip crisp enough to bring from plate to mouth? This version ensures that every chip is evenly covered with protein-packed chicken and fiber-rich beans, plus enough salsa and lime-spiked sour cream to keep your mouth watering.

You'll Need:

- 6 oz tortilla chips (round chips are preferable)
- 1 can (16 oz) black beans, rinsed and drained
- 1½ cups shredded Monterey Jack cheese
- 1 cup shredded chicken (preferably from a store-bought rotisserie chicken)
- ½ red onion, diced

Juice of 2 limes

- ½ cup light sour cream

Chopped cilantro

Salsa (either fresh, page 46, or your favorite bottled salsa)

- Thinly sliced jalapeños (optional)

How to Make It:

- Preheat the oven to 425°F. Arrange the chips in a single layer on a large baking sheet. Spoon the beans evenly over the chips, then top with the cheese, chicken, and onion. Bake for 15 to 20 minutes, until the cheese is fully melted and bubbling. Remove.

- Combine the lime juice, sour cream, and cilantro. Spoon over the nachos. Top with the salsa and jalapeños.

Makes 6 appetizer servings

Want to boost fiber and lower the calorie content? Garden of Eatin' Black Bean are the best tortilla chips in America.

We love pickled jalapeños, which have less bite than raw chiles. Soak jalapeños in white vinegar seasoned with salt and sugar for 30 minutes before serving.

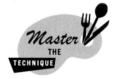

Master THE TECHNIQUE

Nacho Architecture

The secret to a great nacho is balance. Put too much on and that little chip grows soggy and overburdened. Add too little and they're not really nachos, are they? To hit the sweet spot, spread a single layer of chips (the bigger, the better) on a baking sheet. Start with beans, followed by cheese, meats, and vegetables. Save all cold toppings (guac, salsa, etc.) for after the nachos emerge from the oven.

Per Serving

$2.65

330 calories

12 g fat
(6 g saturated)

500 mg sodium

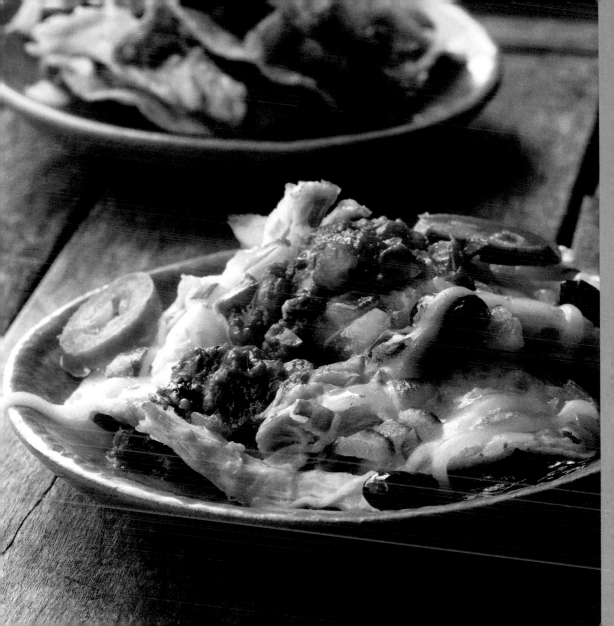

Spinach-Artichoke Dip

This classic dip is normally hijacked by a roguish team of full-fat mayo and cream cheese; somewhere, hidden within, lie token amounts of spinach and artichoke. Here, we turn that ratio on its head, plus use a flavorful olive oil-based mayo to cut calories and boost nutrition. Chiles bring some extra heat to the equation, while toasted wheat pitas work as super scoopers. Overall, this reimagined appetizer packs an amazing 14 grams of fiber.

You'll Need:

- 4 large whole-wheat pitas
- ½ Tbsp butter
- 1 onion, finely chopped
- 3 cloves garlic, finely chopped
- 1 jar (12 oz) artichoke hearts in water, drained and chopped
- 1 box (16 oz) chopped frozen spinach, thawed
- 1 can (4 oz) roasted green chiles, drained and chopped
- 2 Tbsp olive oil mayonnaise (made by both Kraft and Hellmann's)
- 2 Tbsp whipped cream cheese
- Juice of 1 lemon
- Salt and black pepper to taste

How to Make It:

- Cut the pitas into 6 to 8 wedges each and separate the layers. Spread on 2 baking sheets and bake at 400°F for 5 minutes or until crisp.

- Heat the butter in a large skillet or sauté pan over medium heat. Add the onion and garlic and cook for 5 minutes or until softened. Add the artichokes, spinach, chiles, mayonnaise, cream cheese, and lemon juice. Cook, stirring often, for 5 minutes or until hot. Season with salt and pepper. Serve with the pita wedges.

Makes 4 servings

Whipped cream cheese has air beaten into it, making it lighter and easier to spread.

Per Serving
$2.07
270 calories
10 g fat
(2.5 g saturated)
520 mg sodium

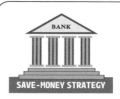

SAVE-MONEY STRATEGY

Fresh spinach generally runs about $3 a bunch, and because spinach is made up of around 90 percent water, it cooks down to nothing as soon as it touches the pan. Frozen spinach not only costs less than half as much as fresh, but also, because it's precooked, yields significantly more actual spinach. Always keep a box in the freezer for this and other recipes that call for cooked spinach.

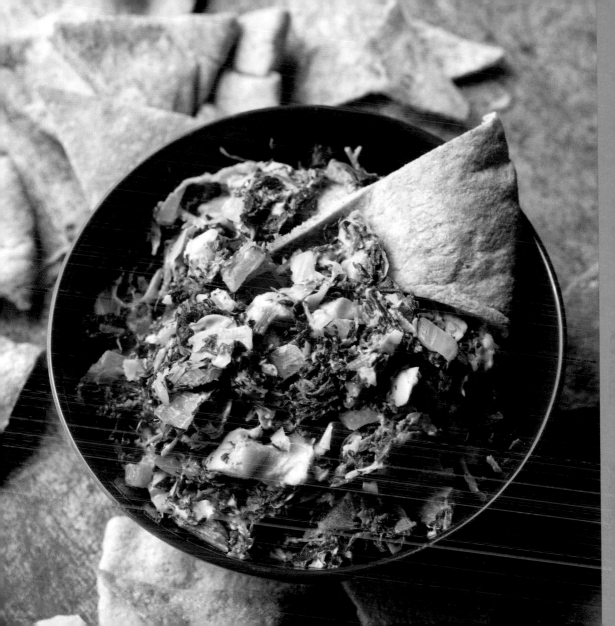

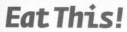
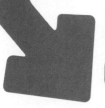

Mexican Shrimp Cocktail

Mexican cuisine is all about the condiments and accoutrements, a philosophy exemplified in sophisticated and humble dishes alike. Take these crustaceans. Whereas Yankee shrimp cocktail consists simply of shrimp and sauce, Mexican palates demand más: cubes of creamy avocado, currents of hot sauce, bright notes of fresh herbs and citrus. It's our favorite kind of move, one that boosts flavor and improves nutrition simultaneously.

You'll Need:

- 1 medium cucumber, peeled, seeded, and chopped
- 1 small red onion, diced
- 1 avocado, pitted, peeled, and chopped
- ¼ cup chopped fresh cilantro
- ½ cup ketchup
- Juice of 2 limes
- 2 Tbsp Mexican hot sauce like Tapatío, Cholula, or Valentina
- 1 tsp Worcestershire sauce
- Salt and black pepper to taste
- 12 oz (51 to 60 count) small cooked shrimp
- Tortilla chips, crackers, or toasted corn tortillas for serving

How to Make It:

- Combine the cucumber, onion, avocado, cilantro, ketchup, lime juice, hot sauce, and Worcestershire in a large mixing bowl. Stir and taste, adjusting the seasoning with salt, pepper, and more hot sauce if needed. Stir in the shrimp and let sit for at least 15 minutes before serving.

- Serve in mason jars, drinking glasses, or wide-mouthed wine glasses (if you want to be a bit fancy) with crackers, chips, or tostadas. Garnish with extra cilantro and avocado if you like.

Makes 4 servings

Saltines are traditional with this dish, but we prefer Triscuits or tostadas. Make tostadas by baking corn tortillas in a 350°F oven for 15 minutes.

Per Serving
$2.84
250 calories
10 g fat
(1 g saturated)
820 mg sodium

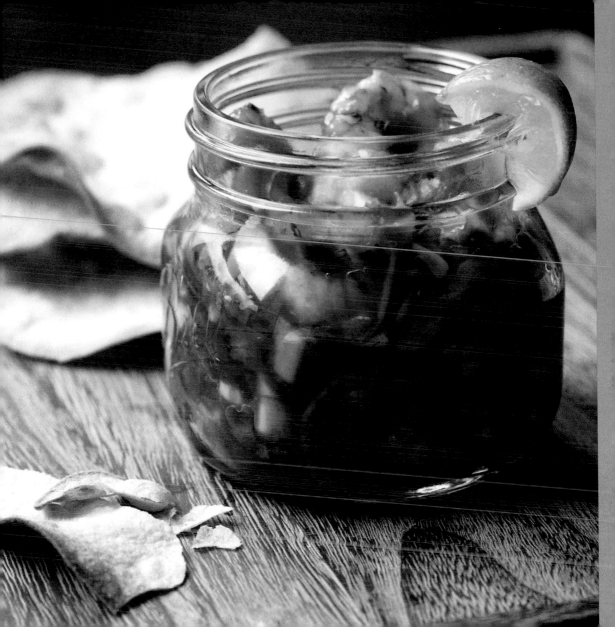

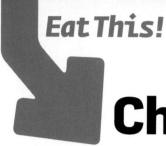

Eat This!

Cheese Fries

When we released our first list of the 20 Worst Foods in America back in 2007, Outback's Aussie Cheese Fries occupied the top slot, packing an outrageous 2,900 calories and 182 grams of fat. While the steakhouse has managed to trim those numbers ever so slightly, the prospect of eating fried potatoes covered in cheese at a restaurant is as dangerous as ever. This easy home version keeps the calories low by baking the potatoes until crisp, applying just the right amount of cheese, and using a few hunks of crumbled bacon and a handful of pickled jalapeños to give the impression of decadence without the four-digit damage.

You'll Need:

2 large russet potatoes, peeled and cut into ¼" fries

1 Tbsp olive oil

1 tsp chili powder

¼ tsp smoked paprika (optional)

Salt and black pepper to taste

1 cup shredded pepper Jack cheese

4 slices bacon, cooked and crumbled

5 scallions, chopped

Pickled jalapeños (see page 72) or fresh jalapeños, thinly sliced

How to Make It:

● Preheat the oven to 425°F. Toss the potatoes with the olive oil, chili powder, smoked paprika (if using), and salt and pepper. Spread out on a rimmed baking sheet and bake for about 20 minutes, until deep brown and crispy on the outside. Top with the cheese, bacon, and scallions, and return to the oven. Bake until the cheese is fully melted and beginning to brown. Garnish with pickled jalapeños.

Makes 4 servings

The cut of the fry is critical. Slice off the lengths of the potato to create flat surfaces, then cut the potato into ¼-inch planks. Stack the planks and cut into ¼-inch fries.

Per Serving
$1.21
300 calories
13 g fat
(5 g saturated)
310 mg sodium

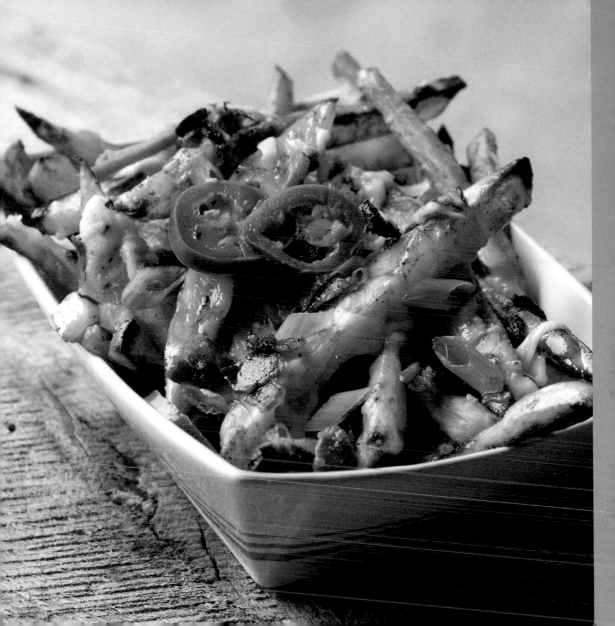

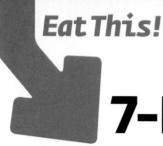

Eat This!

7-Layer Dip

An emerging star in the American potluck scene circa 1985, the seven-story dip has proven to be a surprisingly enduring entertaining staple in the ensuing decades. Most versions pile one packaged good on top of another, resulting in a sludgy industrial stew that grows old after the first bite. This version lightens up matters with spicy ground turkey, fresh pico de gallo, and whole black beans, plus a spoonful of creamy Greek yogurt standing in for sour cream. You can serve this in one giant dish, but building separate layered servings in individual glasses makes for a dramatic presentation and allows for all the double-dipping one could want.

You'll Need:

- 10 corn tortillas, cut into triangles
- 1 Tbsp canola oil
- Salt to taste
- 1 tsp olive oil
- 8 oz ground turkey
- 1 tsp chili powder
- ⅛ tsp cayenne
- Black pepper to taste
- 1 can (15 oz) black beans, drained and rinsed
- Juice of 1 lime
- 1 tsp cumin
- ¼ cup Guacamole (page 320) or store-bought guac
- 1 can (4 oz) diced roasted green chiles
- ½ cup Pico de Gallo (page 319) or store-bought salsa
- ¼ cup 2% Greek yogurt
- ½ cup sliced or chopped black olives

Per Serving
$1.38
280 calories
13 g fat
(2 g saturated)
480 mg sodium

How to Make It:

- Preheat the oven to 425°F. Toss the tortillas with the canola oil and spread out across a baking sheet. (You may need two sheets to keep the chips from overlapping.) Bake for about 10 minutes, until golden brown and crispy. Season with salt once they come out of the oven.

- While the tortillas bake, heat the olive oil in a medium sauté pan over medium heat. Add the turkey and cook for about 5 minutes, until cooked through, seasoning with the chili powder, cayenne, and salt and pepper as it cooks.

- Combine the black beans with the lime juice, cumin, and salt and black pepper to taste.

- In a large ramekin or glass serving dish, build the dip: Spread the guacamole on the bottom, top with the black beans, then the turkey, chiles, pico de gallo, yogurt, and olives. Serve with the tortilla chips.

Makes 6 servings

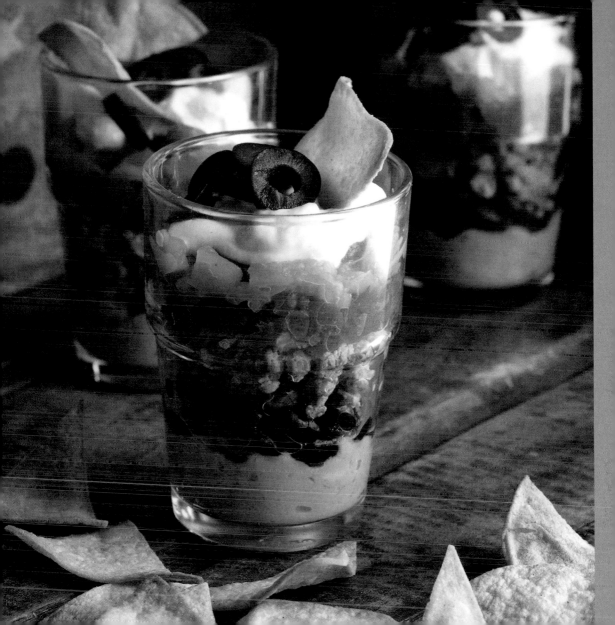

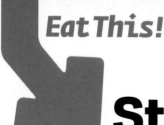

Eat This!

Stuffed Dates

Sometimes it's truly astounding just how little effort it takes to make food taste great. This recipe, as much as any, proves that point. Sweet, salty, smoky, creamy— in a single bite, these tiny packages take you through the highest peaks of flavor country. Show up at a party or a potluck with these little gems and suddenly you— and your dates—will be inundated with invites to swanky soirees all across town.

You'll Need:

8 Medjool dates

8 almonds

¼ cup crumbled blue cheese •

4 strips bacon, cut in half widthwise

Black pepper to taste

Some people are turned off by the funk of blue cheese, but it's nicely tempered here by the sweetness of the fruit and the smoke of the bacon. Still don't love it? Goat cheese and feta are good substitutes.

How to Make It:

● Preheat the oven to 425°F. Using a sharp paring knife, make a slit along the length of a date so that the pocket in the fruit is exposed. Remove the small pit inside the date and replace with an almond. Spoon about ½ table-spoon of blue cheese into the pocket, so that it's tightly stuffed but not overflowing with cheese. Place the date at the bottom of a bacon strip half and roll up as tightly as possible. Secure with a toothpick. Repeat with the remaining 7 dates.

● Place the dates on a nonstick baking sheet and bake for about 20 minutes, until the fat has rendered and the bacon is brown and crispy. Top each with a bit of black pepper and serve.

Makes 4 servings

Per Serving
$1.76
220 calories
7 g fat
(3 g saturated)
300 mg sodium

STEP-BY-STEP

Stuffing dates

Stuffing dates isn't rocket science, as this recipe will teach you. Just be sure to wrap the bacon extra tight, and to only use just enough to cover the date once.

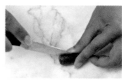

● **STEP 1:** Make a cut across the fruit; scoop out seed.

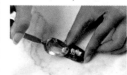

● **STEP 2:** Stuff with almond and a spoonful of cheese.

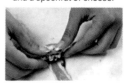

● **STEP 3:** Wrap very tightly with a single layer of bacon.

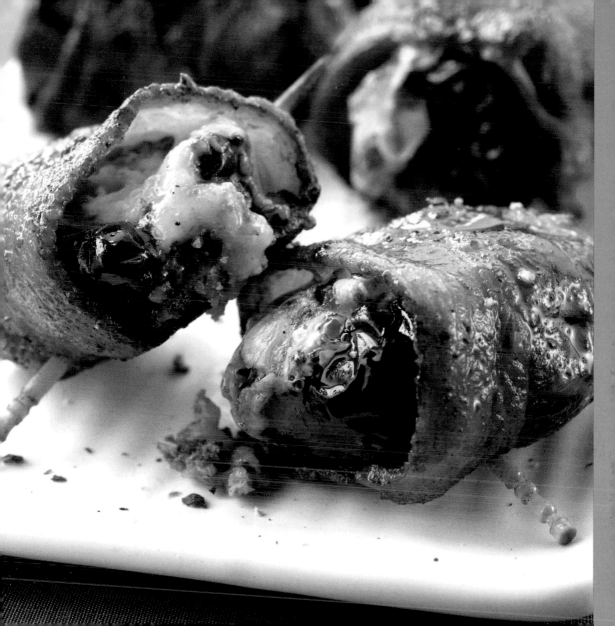

Crispy Quesadillas with Guacamole

Next to nachos, quesadillas are the most perilous food to be found on a Mexican restaurant menu. Overstuffed with cheese and teeming with greasy toppings, quesadillas are all but guaranteed to pack quadruple-digit calories. Our quesadilla reverses the cheese-to-filling ratio, going long on the nutrient-dense vegetables and using just enough chorizo and cheese to make it feel like an indulgence.

You'll Need:

- ½ Tbsp canola oil
- 4 oz chorizo, casing removed
- 1 small red onion, sliced
- 4 oz white button mushrooms, stems removed, sliced
- 1 large poblano pepper, seeded, sliced into thin strips
- Salt and black pepper to taste
- 1½ cups shredded Monterey Jack cheese
- 4 medium whole-wheat tortillas
- Guacamole (see page 320)

How to Make It:

- Heat a large skillet or saute pan over medium-high heat. Add the oil and chorizo; cook until browned, using a wooden spoon to break up the meat into smaller pieces. Remove from the pan and drain all but a thin film of the fat. Return to the heat and add the onion, mushrooms, and pepper; sauté, stirring occasionally, until the vegetables are brown—5 to 7 minutes. Season with salt and black pepper.
- Divide the cheese between 2 tortillas and top each with half of the vegetable mixture. Top with the remaining tortillas.
- Heat a large cast-iron skillet over medium heat. Spray the pan with nonstick cooking spray and cook each quesadilla individually, until the tortillas are brown and crispy and the cheese is fully melted. Cut into 4 or 6 wedges and serve with the guacamole.

Makes 4 servings

Per Serving
$3.11
310 calories
16 g fat
(5 g saturated)
730 mg sodium

SAVVY SHORTCUT

Individually toasting the quesadillas in a cast-iron skillet yields the crispiest, tastiest results imaginable. But if you're making a round for the whole family and want to save time, try the broiler or even the grill (which adds delicious smoky notes to the quesadilla). Simply preheat either, assemble all of your quesadillas, and cook 6" under the broiler or directly on the grill grates for 3 to 4 minutes per side, until toasted on the outside and melted in the middle.

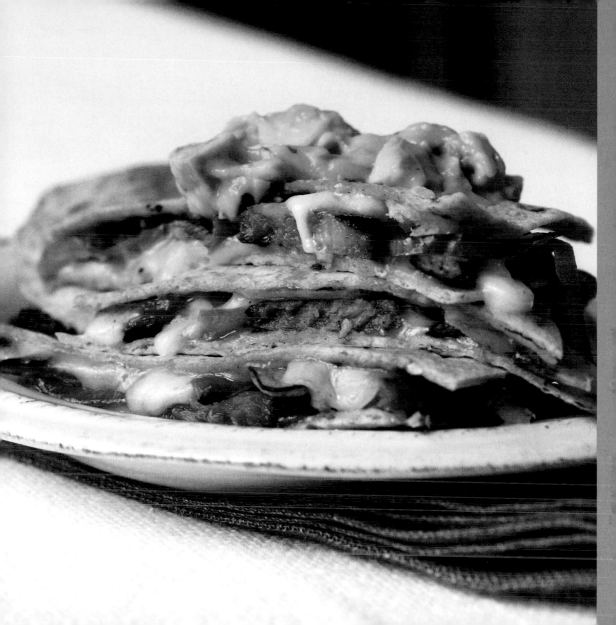

Smoky Deviled Eggs

Have we mentioned our affinity for the egg? Beyond being a near-perfect nutritional substance (think: protein, healthy fat, and vital nutrients like lutein, which protects your eyes from degeneration), no other food is so versatile: It is capable of being fried, poached, baked, boiled, scrambled, and emulsified. And, of course, deviled. It might not be the healthiest way to eat an egg (that honor would go to boiling or poaching), but in terms of snacks and finger foods, it's hard to beat this Southern specialty.

You'll Need:

8 eggs

¼ cup olive oil mayonnaise

½ Tbsp Dijon mustard

2 tsp canned chipotle pepper

Salt and black pepper to taste

Paprika (preferably the smoked Spanish-style paprika called pimenton)

2 strips bacon, cooked and finely crumbled

How to Make It:

● Bring a pot or large saucepan of water to a full boil. Carefully lower the eggs into the water and cook for 8 minutes. Drain and immediately place in a bowl of ice water. When the eggs have cooled, peel them while they're still in the water (the water helps the shell slide off).

● Cut the eggs in half and scoop out the yolks. Combine the yolks with the mayo, mustard, chipotle pepper, and a good pinch each of salt and black pepper. Stir to combine thoroughly. Scoop the mixture into a sealable plastic bag, pushing it all the way into one corner. Cut a small hole in the corner. Squeeze to pipe the yolk mixture back into the whites. Top each with a sprinkle of paprika and a bit of crumbled bacon.

Makes 4 servings

Spanish-style paprika adds more than just a visual pop; it brings a smoky note to the eggs that reinforces the smoke from the bacon and the chipotle.

Per Serving
$0.70
220 calories
17 g fat
(4 g saturated)
370 mg sodium

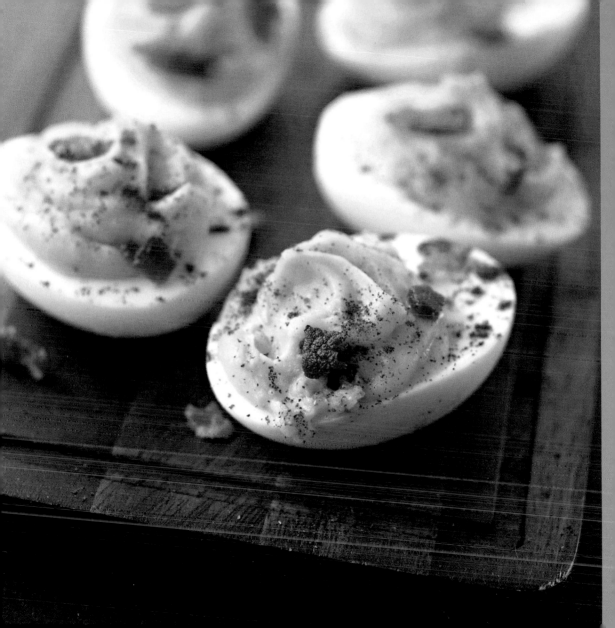

SOUPS
& SALADS

America's Worst SOUPS & SALADS

WORST ONION SOUP
Outback Steakhouse's Too Right French Onion Soup

466 calories
31 g fat
(15 g saturated, 1 g trans)
2,733 mg sodium
Price: $4.99

Sure, this French specialty has some good things going for it—lean beef broth and antioxidant-rich onions—but a generous crowning of melted provolone pretty much cancels out its nutritional merits. Thanks to its cheesy cap, this sinful soup houses three-quarters of your recommended daily saturated fat count, and while 466 calories isn't a terrible load on its own, it's a pitiful prelude to a full entrée.

Eat This Instead!
French Onion Soup
(page 98)

230 calories
8 g fat (4 g saturated)
720 mg sodium
Cost per serving: $2.93
Save! 236 calories and $2.06!

35 grams of saturated fat

Panera sullies soup's good name with this cataclysmic bowl of chowder.

Panera Bread's New England Clam Chowder

630 calories
54 g fat
(35 g saturated, 1.5 g trans)
890 mg sodium
Price: $4.89

New England: home to the skinniest Americans and the fattiest soup. Cream is the caloric culprit here, and it translates to a bowl with nearly two days' worth of saturated fat and more calories than four cans of Campbell's Chicken Noodle. Add to that a hefty dose of hazardous trans fats and you've got the worst liquid lunch in the land. Stick with meat- or vegetable-based broths to ensure your soup doesn't drown your get-slim plans.

Eat This Instead!
Clam Chowder (page 104)

270 calories
6 g fat (2 g saturated)
650 mg sodium
Cost per serving: $2.56
Save! 360 calories and $2.33!

California Pizza Kitchen's Field Greens Salad with Gorgonzola (full)

910 calories
66 g fat (15 g saturated)
973 mg sodium
Price: $11.75

There's not an unhealthy ingredient on this plate: field greens, pears, heart-healthy walnuts, oil-based dressing.

Even the Gorgonzola isn't a terrible salad topper, in moderate doses. And therein lies the problem: There's nothing moderate about the menu at CPK. No matter how nutritious the ingredients, when you serve up a salad in a portion fit for a king, you're going to turn your patrons into pot-bellied paupers. Go halfsies or go home at CPK.

Eat This Instead!
Spinach and Goat Cheese Salad with Apples and Warm Bacon Dressing (page 100)

240 calories
17 g fat (5 g saturated)
640 mg sodium
Cost per serving: $2.13
Save! 670 calories and $9.62!

Applebee's Oriental Chicken Salad

1,390 calories
98 g fat
(15 g saturated, 1.5 g trans)
1,660 mg sodium
Price: $8.99

Topping a salad with chicken fingers is like adding a scoop of Ben & Jerry's to your broccoli. We don't know which evil diet doer okayed this trend, but deep-fried flesh has no place on a bed of greens. At Applebee's, the combo of breaded strips and typical restaurant portion distortion makes for a salad with 420 calories more than the chain's Bacon Cheddar Cheeseburger.

Eat This Instead!
Chinese Chicken Salad (page 106)

380 calories
21 g fat (3.5 g saturated)
650 mg sodium
Cost per serving: $3.30
Save! 1,010 calories and $5.69!

Cheesecake Factory's Cobb Salad

1,550 calories
N/A g fat (26 g saturated)
2,418 mg sodium
Price: $14.95

We're convinced the Cheesecake Factory could turn an organic carrot into a legitimate health liability. There's no surprise, then, that it takes Cobb's traditional combo of eggs, bacon, avocado, and cheese and creates a salad with more calories than most restaurants' worst entrée. At home, you can create all kinds of decadent combinations (like asparagus, prosciutto, and a fried egg!) with none of the flab, but at the Factory, the Skinny-Licious menu is your only hope for staying, well, skinny.

Eat This Instead!
Asparagus with Fried Eggs and Prosciutto (page 110)

260 calories
17 g fat (4 g saturated)
520 mg sodium
Cost per serving: $1.88
Save! 1,290 calories and $13.07!

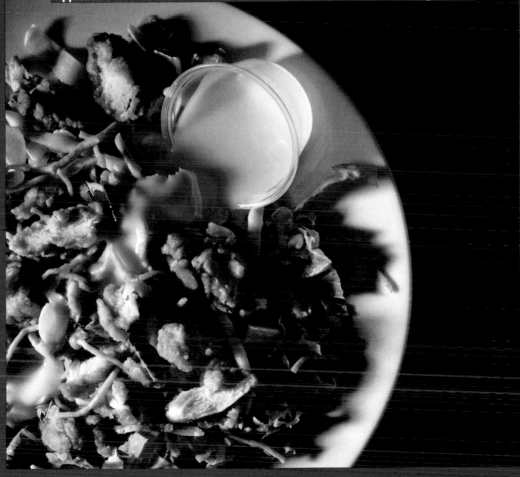

1,390 calories

Applebee's Oriental Chicken Salad: three meals' worth of calories in a single bowl!

Hand Blender

You're lazy. But don't feel bad—we're lazy too. And the more we embrace our laziness, the better we're able to accommodate it. Many of the world's greatest innovations came from the desire to make life easier.

That's where the hand blender (or immersion blender, if you prefer) comes in. It's an instrument of ease, an understated luxury of the kitchen. If you call it the lazy person's blender, then you understand its function. The typical cleaning process amounts to little more than running it under water and stuffing it back into a drawer. Traditional blenders are bulky and messy, but hand blenders are ergonomic and easy to clean. And that makes us lazy people happy.

But there's more. The hand blender does more than just clean up easily; it also makes healthy dishes easier to prepare. Like a traditional blender, the hand blender whirs fruit into smoothies, beans into dips, and ice into the slush of a frozen cocktail. But unlike a traditional blender, you can submerge it directly into almost any vessel—whether a bowl filled with the ingredients for a salad dressing or a hot stockpot loaded with bubbling vegetable soup. If you've tried pouring hot vegetables into a blender jar, then you understand the challenge: The jar becomes painfully hot, and you have to work in several batches to blend the entire soup. Consider the hand blender your no-hassle remedy.

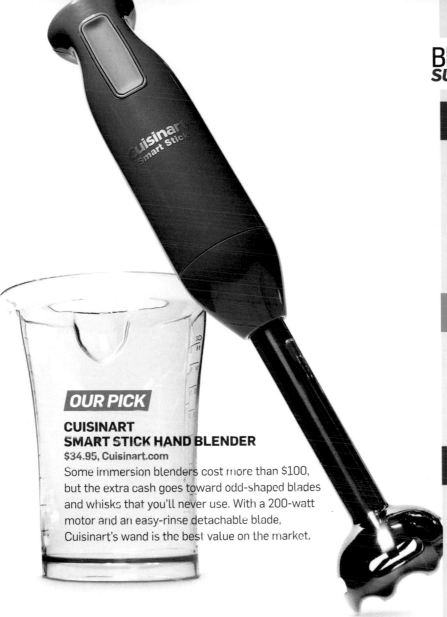

Blender SUPERPOWERS

IMPROVISE SOUPS

For a hot-and-creamy soup, sauté carrots, onions, and celery in a bit of oil, then add your favorite vegetable (mushrooms, butternut squash, potatoes) and plenty of stock or water. Simmer until the vegetables are soft, then drop the blender into the pot and puree. Add salt, pepper, and whatever fresh herbs or spices you have on hand. Swirl in olive oil or yogurt for richer body before serving.

PULVERIZE PESTO

Combine a bunch of basil with 1 clove of garlic, 2 tablespoons pine nuts, ¼ cup grated Parmesan cheese, and ¼ cup olive oil. Blend until you have a smooth emerald-green sauce. Use for dressing pasta or salad, or as a dipping sauce for grilled chicken or fish.

BLEND UP BREAKFAST

A good hand blender can pulverize fruit into a creamy smoothie in a matter of seconds. Remember this ratio: 2 cups fruit (preferably frozen, which makes for a colder, creamier smoothie), ½ cup juice, and ½ cup Greek yogurt.

OUR PICK

CUISINART SMART STICK HAND BLENDER

$34.95, Cuisinart.com

Some immersion blenders cost more than $100, but the extra cash goes toward odd-shaped blades and whisks that you'll never use. With a 200-watt motor and an easy-rinse detachable blade, Cuisinart's wand is the best value on the market.

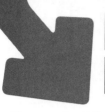

Eat This!

Mom's Chicken Noodle Soup

Curer of colds, warmer of hearts, soother of souls: Chicken noodle soup does everything a comfort food is supposed to do, and does so without a hefty caloric price tag. But steer clear of canned chicken soup: Not only is it sparse on chicken and vegetables, a single cup can carry up to half a day's worth of sodium. This version is light on the salt, but so loaded with chunky vegetables and shredded chicken that it could be dinner on its own.

You'll Need:

- ½ Tbsp olive oil
- 3 medium carrots, peeled and chopped
- 3 ribs celery, chopped
- 1 small onion, chopped
- 1 clove garlic, peeled
- 12 cups low-sodium chicken stock
- 1 bay leaf
- 2 cups shredded leftover chicken
- 2 oz dried egg noodles

Salt and black pepper to taste

Chopped fresh parsley for garnish (optional)

How to Make It:

- Heat the olive oil in a pot over medium heat. Add the carrots, celery, onion, and garlic and sauté for 5 minutes, until the vegetables just begin to soften. Add the stock and bay leaf and cook over low heat for about 15 minutes, until the carrots are just tender.

- Add the chicken and noodles and continue cooking for about 5 minutes, just until the noodles are soft. Taste and adjust seasoning with salt and black pepper if necessary. Discard the bay leaf and garlic clove. Garnish with parsley before serving, if using.

Makes 6 servings

Per Serving
$1.86
225 calories
4 g fat
(1 g saturated)
720 mg sodium

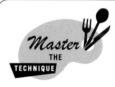

Master **THE** `TECHNIQUE`

Homemade Chicken Stock

Store-bought stock works just fine for every recipe in the book, but nothing compares to the flavor of a home-cooked batch. Combine scraps of chicken (back, wings, even bones from a roast chicken) with a mirepoix (onions, carrots, and celery) and herbs (bay leaf and parsley), cover with plenty of water, and simmer for an hour. Add depth by mixing in garlic, mushrooms, or even a bit of tomato paste before simmering.

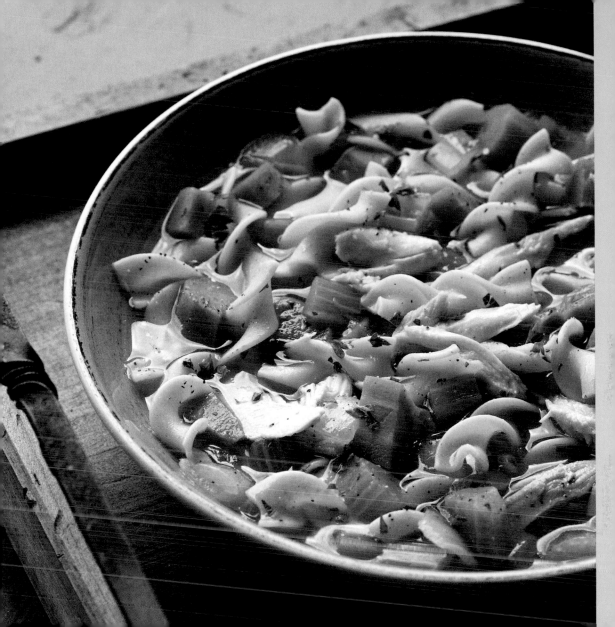

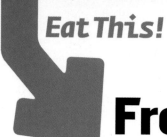

Eat This!

French Onion Soup

We're not going to lie: Good French onion soup takes time. But it takes almost no effort, other than fighting back the tears as you chop your way through the five onions. And wouldn't you rather deal with a few errant tears than with a lackluster, overpriced bowl of soup that packs as much saturated fat as 20 strips of bacon and more sodium than nine bags of Lay's potato chips? (Don't believe us? Check out page 90.) Now that's a real reason to cry.

You'll Need:

- 1 Tbsp butter
- 5 medium onions (a mix of yellow and red is ideal), sliced
- ½ tsp salt
- 2 bay leaves
- 6 cups low-sodium beef broth
- ½ cup dry red wine
- 4 or 5 sprigs fresh thyme (optional)
- Freshly cracked pepper
- 4 slices baguette or sourdough bread
- ½ cup shredded Swiss cheese

Chicken and vegetable broths are fine, too, but beef broth is best for bringing out the rich meatiness of the onions.

How to Make It:

- Heat the butter in a large pot over low heat. Add the onions and salt. Cover the pot and cook the onions over low heat until very soft and caramelized, about 30 minutes. (Most of this is unsupervised. Check on the onions and stir every 10 minutes or so.)
- Add the bay leaves, broth, wine, and thyme (if using). Simmer on low heat for at least 15 minutes. Season with pepper. Discard the bay leaves.
- Preheat the broiler. Divide the soup among 4 oven-proof bowls. Top each with a slice of baguette and some cheese. Broil until the cheese is melted and bubbling, about 3 minutes.

Makes 4 servings

Per Serving
$2.93
230 calories
8 g fat
(4 g saturated)
720 mg sodium

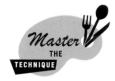

Master THE **TECHNIQUE**

Precision salting

Salt comes in dozens of shapes, sizes, and colors, but really it all comes down to three varieties: iodized salt (fine salt for use at the table), flaky sea salt (its crunchy texture is best used on cooked dishes like grilled steak and fish), and, most important, kosher salt. Chefs use kosher salt to season dishes as they're cooking because the coarse crystals allow them to season with precision. You should do the same, always using your hands (never a shaker!) to season.

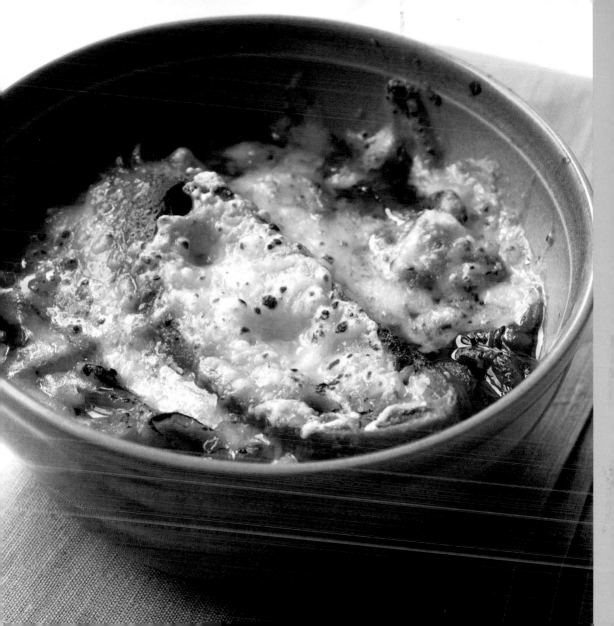

Eat This!

Spinach & Goat Cheese Salad
with Apples & Warm Bacon Dressing

We love the idea of wilted spinach (especially if it's bacon drippings doing the wilting!), but this old standby needs some updating. A great salad should be many things: sweet and salty, crunchy and tender—a full exploration of taste and texture. With the addition of caramelized apples, toasted pecans, and creamy goat cheese, this retro spinach salad finally achieves perfect harmony in the 21st century.

You'll Need:

- 6 strips bacon, chopped
- 1 small red onion, sliced
- 1 green apple, peeled and sliced
- ¼ cup pecans
- 2 Tbsp red wine vinegar
- 1 Tbsp Dijon mustard
- 1 Tbsp olive oil
- Salt and black pepper to taste
- 1 bunch spinach, washed, dried, and stemmed
- ¼ cup fresh goat cheese

How to Make It:

- Heat a large cast-iron skillet or nonstick pan over medium heat. Add the bacon and cook for about 5 minutes, until browned and just crisp. Remove to a paper towel–lined plate and reserve.

- Add the onion to the same pan and cook for 2 to 3 minutes, until just soft. Add the apple and pecans and continue sautéing for 2 minutes, until the pecans are lightly toasted and the apple softened. Add the vinegar, mustard, and olive oil, along with a few pinches of salt and plenty of black pepper. Use a wooden spoon to stir the mixture vigorously to help it emulsify into a unified dressing.

- Divide the spinach and goat cheese among 4 bowls and pour the warm dressing directly over the greens. Garnish with the reserved bacon.

Makes 4 servings

Per Serving
$2.13
240 calories
17 g fat
(5 g saturated)
640 mg sodium

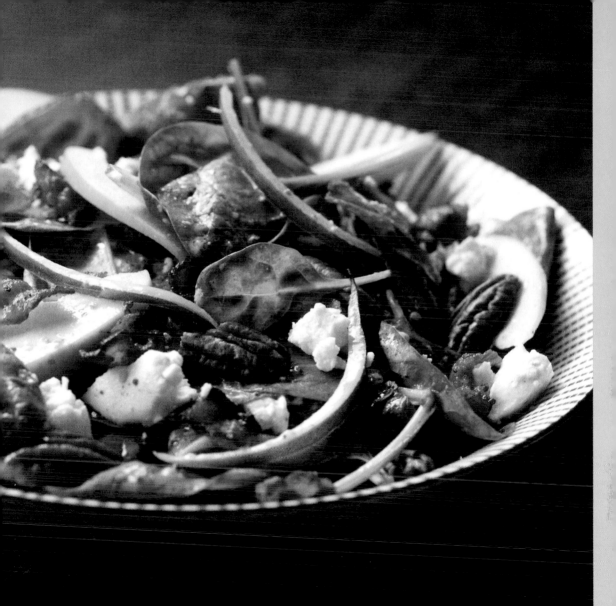

Italian Sausage Soup

The best definition of comfort food is the food Mom made when you were growing up. Matt's mom made Italian sausage soup, a deceptively simple but wonderfully soothing bowl of meat, vegetables, and pasta—like chicken soup for the Italian soul. You can load this one full of vegetables, doubling the amount used below, and end up with a chunky, sausage-strewn minestrone. Either way, this soup is hearty enough to work as dinner on its own.

You'll Need:

- ½ Tbsp olive oil
- 2 links Italian-style turkey sausage, casings removed
- 1 small yellow onion, diced
- 2 cloves garlic, minced
- Pinch of red pepper flakes
- 1 can (14 oz) diced tomatoes
- 8 cups low-sodium chicken broth
- ¾ cup farfalle, preferably whole wheat, or other pasta
- 2 cups green beans, tips removed, halved
- Parmesan for serving

How to Make It:

- Heat the olive oil in a large saucepan or pot over medium heat. Add the sausage meat and cook for 3 to 5 minutes, until no longer pink. Transfer to a plate and reserve.
- Add the onion, garlic, and red pepper flakes to the same pot and cook for about 5 minutes, until the onion is soft. Add the tomatoes and chicken broth and bring to a low boil. Stir in the pasta, cook for 6 minutes, then add the green beans and the reserved sausage. Simmer for about 5 minutes longer, just until the pasta is cooked through and the beans are soft. Serve with grated Parmesan.

Makes 4 servings

A few cups of baby spinach or chopped broccoli would work as a substitute for the green beans.

Per Serving
$2.39
360 calories
12 g fat
(2.5 g saturated)
890 mg sodium

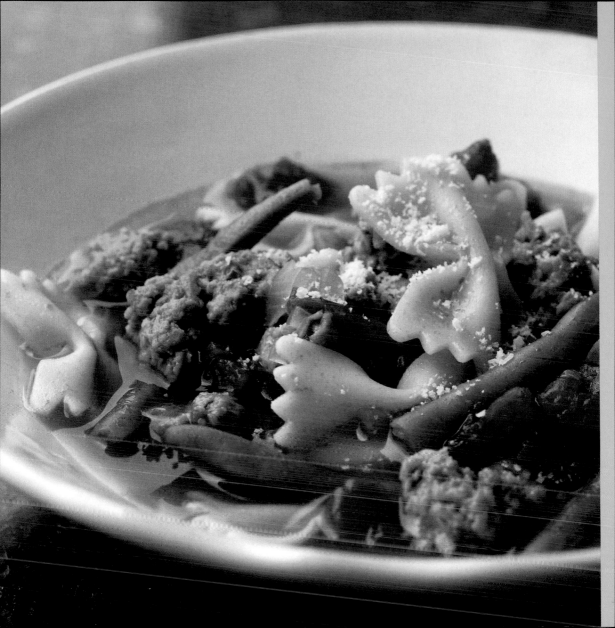

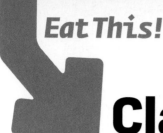

Clam Chowder

Most people expect a bowl of soup so thick and creamy you can stand a spoon up in it, but truth is, clam chowder, real clam chowder, has always been about the clams, with a thin but bracing broth of clam juice and a hit of dairy. We chose milk, which makes a light, clean, low-calorie chowder that won't sit in your stomach all afternoon. There is, however, one item we won't compromise on: bacon, whose smoky flavor pairs perfectly with the brine of the clams. You don't need much—just one strip per serving.

You'll Need:

- 4 strips bacon, chopped
- 1 small onion, diced
- 2 ribs celery, diced
- 1 Tbsp flour
- 1 can (6.5 oz) clams, drained, juices reserved
- 2 cups clam juice
- 1 cup milk
- 2 medium Yukon gold potatoes, peeled and diced (about 1½ cups)
- 2 branches fresh thyme (optional)

Salt and black pepper to taste

How to Make It:

- Cook the bacon in a large saucepan or pot over medium heat for about 5 minutes, until browned and crispy. Transfer to a paper towel–lined plate and reserve.

- Add the onions and celery to the bacon fat and cook for about 5 minutes, until soft. Stir in the flour and cook for 1 minute to eliminate that raw flour taste. Pour in the reserved juices from the clams, the bottled clam juice, and the milk, stirring steadily to ensure the flour is evenly incorporated.

- Bring the mixture to a simmer and add the potatoes and thyme, if using. Simmer for about 10 minutes, just until the potatoes are tender. Season with salt and black pepper. Just before serving, add the clams and simmer long enough to heat them through. Garnish with the reserved bacon.

Makes 4 servings

Per Serving
$2.56
270 calories
6 g fat
(2 g saturated)
650 mg sodium

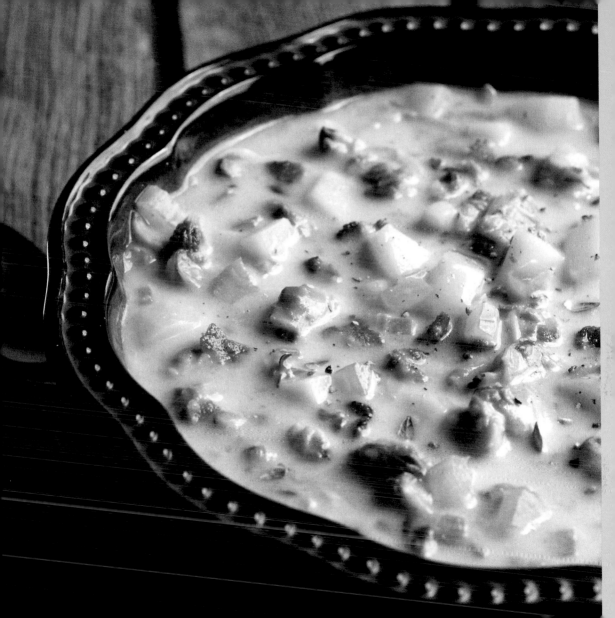

Eat This!

Chinese Chicken Salad

This salad is one of the world's ultimate fusion foods. It's an Eastern-inspired dish popularized by an Austrian chef (Wolfgang Puck) in Beverly Hills (at his restaurant Spago back in the 1980s). Whatever its disparate origins, it's undeniably one of the most popular salads in America, sharing space on menus in four-star restaurants and Wendy's alike. Too bad most versions are nutritional disasters, bogged down by too much dressing and too many fried noodles. This lighter version is true to Wolfgang's original creation.

You'll Need:

- 1 head napa cabbage
- ½ head red cabbage
- ½ Tbsp sugar
- 2 cups chopped or shredded cooked chicken (freshly grilled or from a store-bought rotisserie chicken)
- ⅓ cup Asian-style dressing, like Annie's Shiitake and Sesame Vinaigrette
- 1 cup fresh cilantro leaves
- 1 cup canned mandarin oranges, drained
- ¼ cup sliced almonds, toasted
- Salt and black pepper to taste

How to Make It:

- Slice the cabbages in half lengthwise and remove the cores. Slice the cabbage into thin strips. Toss with the sugar in a large bowl.
- If the chicken is cold, toss with a few tablespoons of vinaigrette and heat in a microwave at 50% power. Add to the cabbage, along with the cilantro, mandarins, almonds, and the remaining vinaigrette. Toss to combine. Season with salt and pepper.

Makes 4 servings

Make sure the mandarins are stored in water, not syrup. You don't want high-fructose corn syrup in your salad, do you?

Per Serving
$3.30
380 calories
21 g fat
(3.5 saturated)
23 g carbs

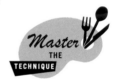

Master THE **TECHNIQUE**

Properly dressing salads

Most salads end up overdressed, which compromises the flavor and the inherent nutritional value of the creation. For a properly dressed salad, add the dressing a few tablespoons at a time immediately before serving (otherwise the lettuce will wilt) and use a pair of tongs to thoroughly distribute each new addition. Pluck a leaf and taste; it should have a light sheen, not a heavy coat, of dressing.

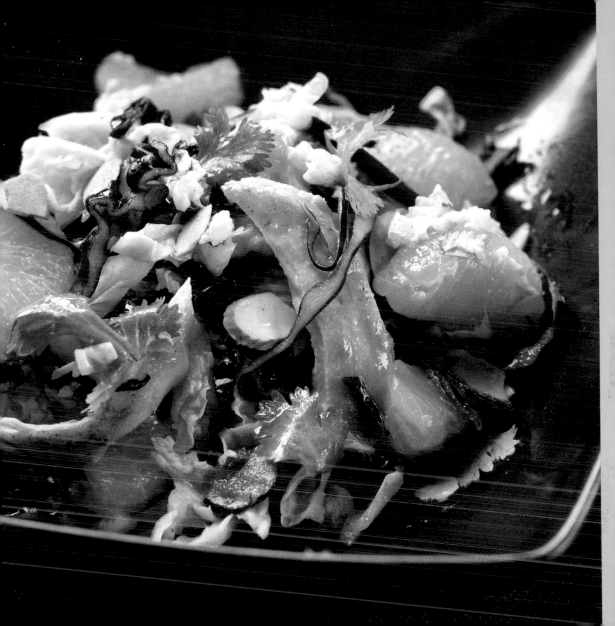

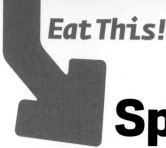

Split Pea Soup

Split peas rank up there as one of the heroes of the health-food world, boasting deep reserves of fiber, B vitamins, and dozens of other vital nutrients. But despite their reputation as a straightlaced superfood, something magical happens to split peas when combined with a bit of smoky ham and a long, slow simmer. Slowly they begin to break down, commingling with the ham and the other vegetables to create a thick, creamy broth that could warm even the most frigid soul on a long winter day.

You'll Need:

- 1 tsp olive oil
- 2 ribs celery, diced
- 1 small onion, diced
- 2 medium carrots, peeled and diced
- 2 cloves garlic, minced
- 10 cups water or low-sodium chicken or vegetable stock
- 2 medium red potatoes, peeled and diced
- 1 smoked ham hock
- 1 cup split peas
- 2 bay leaves

  Salt and black pepper to taste

  Tabasco to taste (optional)

How to Make It:

- Heat the olive oil in a large saucepan or pot over medium heat. Add the celery, onion, carrots, and garlic and sauté for about 5 minutes, until the vegetables are soft. Add the water or stock, the potatoes, ham hock, split peas, and bay leaves. Turn the heat down to low and simmer for about 40 minutes, until the peas have turned very soft and begin to lose their shape, leaving you with a thick soup. (Thin out with more water or stock if you prefer a thinner consistency.)
- Remove the ham hock, shred the meat clinging to the bone, and add back to the soup. Discard the bay leaves. Season to taste with salt and pepper, plus a few shakes of Tabasco, if you like.

Makes 6 servings

Per Serving
$1.24
300 calories
3.5 g fat
(1 g saturated)
780 mg sodium

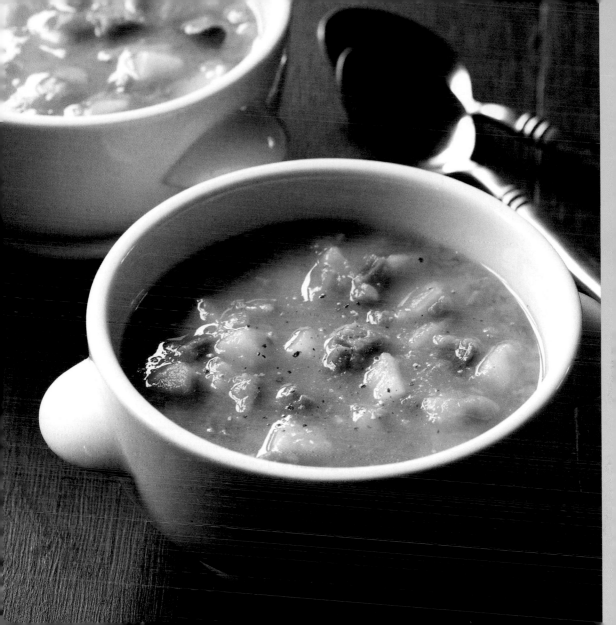

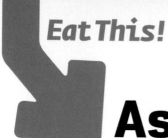

Eat This!

Asparagus with Fried Eggs and Prosciutto

Get it out of your head now that salads are limited to bowls of lettuce. Sturdy vegetables like green beans, broccoli, zucchini, and asparagus can all play the role of a salad foundation every bit as brilliantly as romaine or iceberg. The payoff, as seen so vividly in this dish, is textural contrast: the gentle snap of the asparagus, the creaminess of the soft egg yolk, the crunch of the toasted bread crumbs. This can be a warm-up to dinner (especially if you have guests over), or a light meal on its own.

You'll Need:

- 1 bunch asparagus, woody ends removed
- 3 Tbsp olive oil
- 4 large eggs
- ½ cup homemade bread crumbs (see note)
- 4 slices prosciutto, cut into thin strips
- 2 Tbsp balsamic vinegar
- Coarse sea salt and black pepper to taste

How to Make It:

- Bring a large pot of water to a boil and season with a healthy pinch of salt. Add the asparagus and cook for 3 to 4 minutes, until just tender. Drain and run under cold water to stop the cooking process (which will also help preserve asparagus color).
- Heat 1 tablespoon of the oil in a large nonstick sauté pan. Crack the eggs into the pan and cook for about 5 minutes, just until the whites are set but the yolks are still loose.
- Divide the asparagus among 4 plates. Top each serving with a fried egg and scatter with bread crumbs and prosciutto strips. Drizzle with the remaining olive oil and the vinegar and season with salt and black pepper.

Makes 4 servings

Per Serving
$1.88
260 calories
17 g fat
(4 g saturated)
520 mg sodium

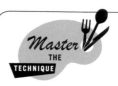

Master THE **TECHNIQUE**

Homemade Bread Crumbs

Store-bought bread crumbs are fine for coating chicken or as binding in meatballs, but to add texture and flavor to salads, soups, and pastas, make your own: Remove the crust from an old loaf of bread and tear the interior into pebble-size pieces. Heat a bit of oil in a pan and cook the bread for about 5 minutes, until golden brown and toasted. For an extra layer of flavor, add whole cloves of garlic or fresh herbs to flavor the cooking oil.

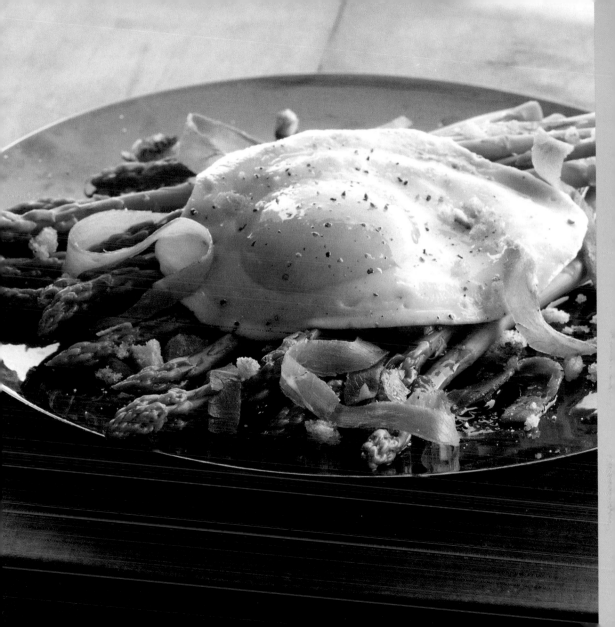

Italian Meatball Soup

Order a plate of spaghetti and meatballs in Italy and you'll likely leave your waiter dumbfounded, scratching his head for an answer. That's because one of America's favorite Italian dishes is a purely American invention, one that generally hinges on our typical tenets of excess. In Italy, polpettine are more likely to be enjoyed in a lighter fashion, either by themselves or in a soup like the one below. The pasta is still there (albeit a much smaller portion of it), but the broth houses a handful of stellar vegetables and serves to keep the meatballs moist and luscious. Though it's light in calories, this is still a potent bowl of goodness—served with a lightly dressed salad, it makes for an incredible weekday dinner.

You'll Need:

- 1 lb ground beef
- 2 medium eggs or 1 extra-large egg
- ¼ cup bread crumbs
- ½ cup finely grated Parmesan cheese
- Salt and ground black pepper to taste
- ½ Tbsp olive oil
- 1 onion, chopped
- 2 carrots, peeled and chopped
- 2 ribs celery, chopped
- 8 cups low-sodium chicken stock
- 1 head escarole, chopped into bite-size pieces
- ¾ cup small pasta, like orzo, pastina, or spaghetti broken into ½-inch pieces

How to Make It:

- Combine the beef with the eggs, bread crumbs, cheese, and good-size pinches of salt and pepper in a mixing bowl. Being careful not to overwork the mixture, lightly form it into meatballs roughly ¾-inch in diameter, a bit smaller than a golf ball.

- Heat the olive oil in a large pot over medium-high heat. Add the onion, carrots, and celery and sauté until the vegetables have softened, about 5 minutes. Add the stock and the escarole and bring the soup to a simmer. Turn the heat down to low and add the meatballs and pasta. Simmer for another 8 to 10 minutes, until the meatballs are cooked through and the pasta is al dente. Taste and adjust the seasoning with salt and pepper.

- Serve the soup with extra cheese on top.

Makes 6 servings

Per Serving
$2.63
333 calories
14 g fat
(5 g saturated)
690 mg sodium

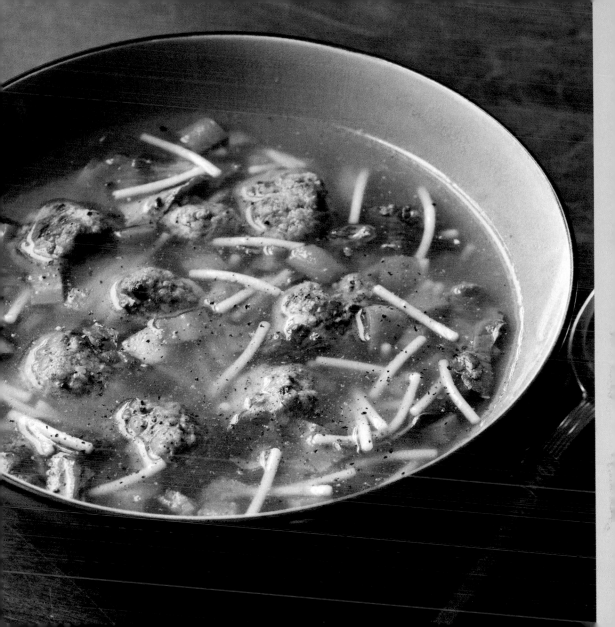

Grilled Cheese & Tomato Soup

An oozing grilled cheese and a cup of warm tomato soup constitute one of the great one-two combos of the comfort food world. Our grilled cheese is a play on that gooey Southern staple, pimento cheese, which diffuses the calories of the cheese with healthy additions like roasted peppers and Greek yogurt. The soup? Pure tomato intensity, thanks to the oven roasting, which concentrates the natural sugars of the tomatoes.

GRILLED PIMENTO CHEESE SANDWICH

You'll Need:

1¼ cups finely shredded sharp Cheddar cheese

1 jar (4 oz) diced pimentos

1 jalapeño pepper, seeded and minced

¼ cup finely sliced scallions

¼ cup 2% Greek yogurt

1 Tbsp olive-oil mayonnaise

Few shakes Tabasco

8 slices bread

Butter

How to Make It:

- Combine the cheese, pimentos, jalapeño, scallions, yogurt, mayonnaise, and a few shakes of Tabasco in a mixing bowl. Divide among 4 slices of bread and top with the remaining slices.

- Heat a bit of butter in a cast-iron skillet or non-stick pan over medium heat. Cook the sandwiches, turning once, for about 10 minutes, until golden brown on both sides and the cheese is melted (have patience—an extra minute or two means everything with good grilled cheese!).

Makes 4 servings

Per Serving
$1.46
320 calories
17 g fat
(8 g saturated)
490 mg sodium

ROASTED TOMATO SOUP

You'll Need:

3 lbs Roma tomatoes, halved lengthwise

2 Tbsp olive oil, plus more for drizzling

4 cloves garlic, peeled

3 cups low-sodium chicken stock

Salt and black pepper to taste

How to Make It:

- Preheat the oven to 425°F. Place the tomatoes cut side up on a baking sheet and drizzle with olive oil. Place the garlic cloves in the center of a sheet of aluminum foil, drizzle with olive oil, and fold to create an enclosed packet.

- Roast the tomatoes and the garlic for about 40 minutes, until both are very soft. Transfer the tomatoes and garlic to a blender, add the olive oil, and puree. Transfer to a pot, stir in the chicken stock, and simmer for 15 minutes. Season with salt and black pepper.

Makes 4 servings

Per Serving
$1.67
130 calories
7 g fat
(1 g saturated)
370 mg sodium

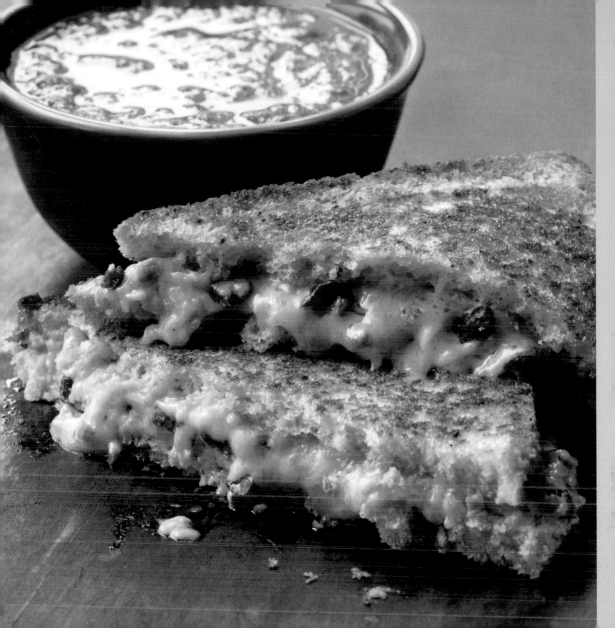

CHAPTER 5

BURGERS & SANDWICHES

America's Worst BURGERS & SANDWICHES

Ruby Tuesday's Avocado Turkey Burger

1,266 calories
67 g fat (15g saturated)
3,216 mg sodium
Price: $9.49

Choosing whole-wheat over white, or grilled over fried, will automatically up your meal's nutritional game, but opting for bird over bovine doesn't always offer the same performance boost. A burger's only as good as its meat, and at Tuesday's, a fatty turkey cut and greasy toppers like bacon and cheese make for a bird burger with more calories than the Classic Cheeseburger. Our turkey burger may be tricked out, but the turkey is lean and the supporting cast is loaded with first-rate side-kicks like fresh avocado and chunky tomato salsa.

Eat This Instead!
Southwest Turkey Burger
(page 136)

470 calories
26 g fat (7 g saturated)
520 mg sodium
Cost per serving: $2.88

Save! 796 calories and $6.61!

118

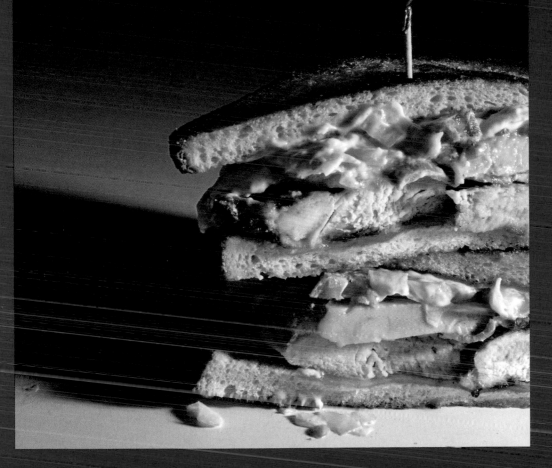

1,750 calories

Only the Cheesecake Factory can turn chicken and avocado into America's Worst Sandwich.

T.G.I. Friday's Whiskey-Glazed Chicken Sandwich

1,110 calories
57 g fat (21g saturated)
2,910 mg sodium
Price: $8.09

You walk into a place like Friday's and you can smell trouble in the air. So you play it safe and order the chicken sandwich. After all, who could screw up a chicken sandwich? Despite your best intentions, you just saddled yourself with as many calories as a Triple Whopper, and more sodium than you should take in over 2 days. Just goes to show that no sandwich is safe—except, of course, the one you make yourself.

Eat This Instead!
Buffalo Chicken & Blue Cheese Sandwich (page 128)

387 calories
15 g fat (5 g saturated)
912 mg sodium
Cost per serving: $3.81
Save! 723 calories and $4.28!

Chili's Jalapeño Smokehouse Burger

1,270 calories
80 g fat (30g saturated)
2,630 mg sodium
Price: $8.79

The *ETNT* Law of Menu Name—Calorie Correlation states that the longer the name of a dish, the more po-tential for nutritional calamity. By that token, Chili's Big Mouth burgers are more than a mouthful. The entire line is littered with sky-high calorie, fat, and sodium counts, thanks to a penchant for overloading the burgers with four or five high-calorie condiments. If you want to get creative with a burger, make sure you're the one doing the creating.

Eat This Instead!
Swiss Burger with Red Wine Mushrooms (page 140)

390 calories
13 g fat (5 g saturated)
360 mg sodium
Cost per serving: $1.90
Save! 880 calories and $6.89!

Jersey Mike's Giant Philly Cheesesteak)

1,270 calories
42.5 g fat (22 g saturated)
3,635 mg sodium
Price: $12.95

No one expects a cheesesteak to be healthy, but few expect a simple lunch to pack more sodium than a dozen large orders of McDonald's french fries. This hero's fatal flaw? Excess. From the jumbo roll, to the bulge of beef, to the sea of oily cheese sauce, it will take a snake jaw, elastic pants, and two packs of Alka-Selzter to put this thing away.

Eat This Instead!
Philly Cheesesteak (page 126)

540 calories
25 g fat (10 g saturated)
790 mg sodium
Cost per serving: $3.93
Save! 730 calories and $9.02!

Cheesecake Factory's Grilled Chicken and Avocado Club

1,220 calories
N/A g fat (22 g saturated)
1,765 mg sodium
Price: $12.95

The club is a simple sand-wich—meat, lettuce, tomato, and mayo between three slices of toast—but no place turns simple into sinful quite like the Cheesecake Factory. We're not sure how the chain was able turn grilled chicken and avocado into a sandwich worse than its worst burger, but we're guessing it has something to do with butter-drenched toast, globs of mayo, piles of bacon, and general Factory tomfoolery. Do you really want to pay $13 for a sandwich that eats up nearly an entire day's worth of calories? Didn't think so.

Eat This Instead!
Ultimate Club Sandwich with Super Mayo (page 130)

330 calories
12 g fat (2.5 g saturated)
980 mg sodium
Cost per serving: $2.68
Save! 890 calories and $10.27!

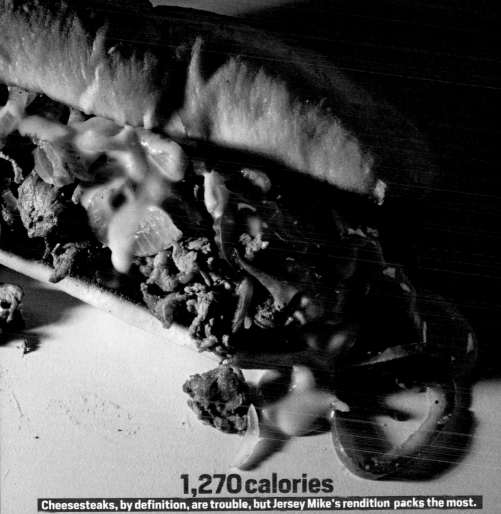

1,270 calories

Cheesesteaks, by definition, are trouble, but Jersey Mike's rendition packs the most.

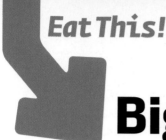

Bigger Better Mac

We're big fans of the Big Mac (after all, it was on the cover of the first *Eat This, Not That!* book)—or at least the general principle behind it. The thin patties, the layer of American cheese, the special sauce, all of it comes together in a way that makes this burger a convincing icon of the American fast-food establishment. But there are two main issues with the Mac as it stands: The quality of the ingredients is subpar and the middle bun is absolutely superfluous. We replace the mystery meat with lean ground sirloin, sear it in a cast-iron skillet until beautifully browned, then bring the classic ingredients together inside a single, squishy sesame seed bun.

You'll Need:

- 2 Tbsp olive-oil mayonnaise
- 1 Tbsp mustard
- 1 Tbsp ketchup
- 1 Tbsp grated onion
- 1 Tbsp sweet pickle relish
- 1 tsp Worcestershire sauce
- 1 lb ground sirloin

Salt and black pepper to taste

- 4 slices American cheese
- 8 dill pickle slices
- ½ cup minced yellow onion
- 4 sesame seed buns, lightly toasted
- 1 cup shredded iceberg lettuce

How to Make It:

- To make the special sauce, in a mixing bowl, combine the mayonnaise, mustard, ketchup, grated onion, relish, and Worcestershire.
- Form the beef into 8 even balls. Use your hands or a spatula to flatten the balls into thin patties on a cutting board.
- Preheat a large cast-iron skillet over medium-high heat. Season the patties on both sides with salt and black pepper. When very hot, add 4 of the patties to the skillet. Cook for about 1 minute, until a brown crust develops. Flip, cover 2 of the patties with a slice of cheese, and continue cooking for 60 to 90 seconds longer, until the bottoms also have a crust. Top each cheeseburger with 2 pickles and a handful of minced onion. Stack the naked burgers on top of the cheeseburgers and remove to a cutting board. Repeat with the remaining 4 patties.
- Spread the bun bottoms with a generous amount of special sauce and top with shredded lettuce. Place the burgers on the buns, top with the bun tops, and serve.

Makes 4 servings

Per Serving
$2.46
380 calories
15 g fat
(5 g saturated)
760 mg sodium

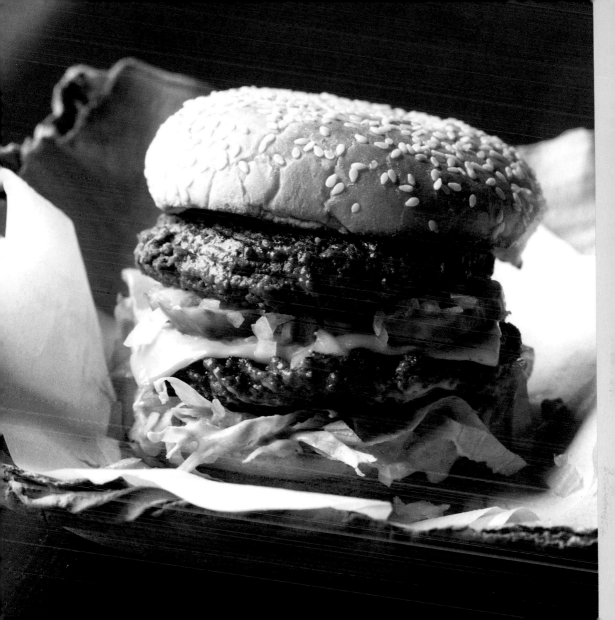

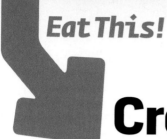

Eat This!

Croque Monsieur

Think of a croque monsieur as a ham and cheese sandwich on steroids: The ham is sliced thick, the cheese—intensely nutty Gruyère—comes melted in a blanket of béchamel, and the whole package is served browned and bubbling straight from the oven. Normally the result is a bilevel calorie bonanza, but this one, a single-layer knife-and-fork affair, delivers on the decadence without the excess calories. Serve with a spinach and apple salad and a glass of red wine for a weeknight dinner that will take the sting out of the workday.

You'll Need:

- 1 Tbsp butter
- 1 Tbsp flour
- 1 cup low-fat milk
- ½ cup shredded Gruyère or other Swiss cheese
- Pinch of grated nutmeg
- Salt and black pepper to taste
- 4 tsp Dijon mustard
- 4 thick slices country bread, lightly toasted
- 8 oz Black Forest ham in 8 slices

How to Make It:

- Preheat the broiler.
- Melt the butter in a medium saucepan over medium heat. Stir in the flour and cook, stirring, until golden brown. Add the milk, whisking to prevent any lumps from forming. Simmer for 5 minutes, until the sauce thickens, then stir in the cheese. Cook the béchamel for another few minutes, until the cheese is evenly melted, then season with nutmeg and salt and pepper.
- Spread a teaspoon of mustard on each piece of bread, then top with the ham. Place on a baking sheet, then ladle on the béchamel. Place the baking sheet on the middle rack and broil for about 5 minutes, until the béchamel is bubbling and nicely browned.

Makes 4 servings

Per Serving
$1.90
410 calories
12 g fat
(6 g saturated)
870 mg sodium

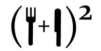

MEAL MULTIPLIER

Knife-and-fork sandwiches achieve the impossible feat of feeling more substantial while actually being lighter. Follow the same broiling technique here for any of these combinations:

- Roast turkey, Apple-Sausage Stuffing (page 304), gravy
- Garlic-Rosemary Roast Beef (page 208), caramelized onions, spicy mustard, provolone cheese
- Roasted vegetables, pesto, fresh mozzarella

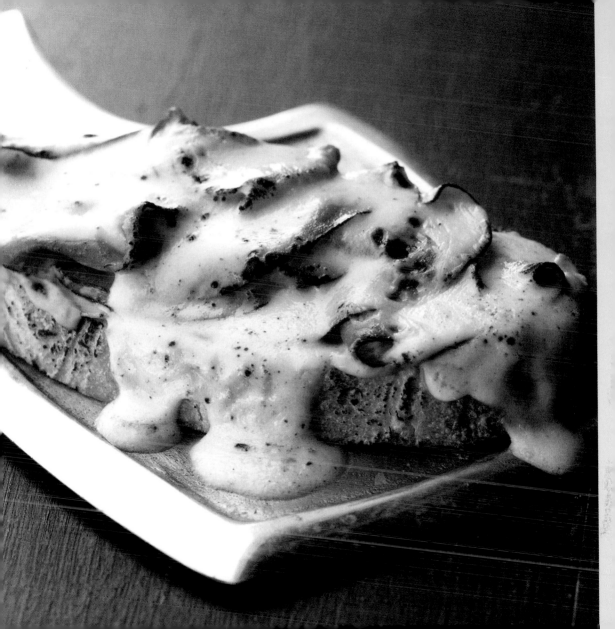

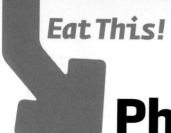

Philly Cheesesteak

Philadelphia is Sandwich Town USA, home to the Italian hoagie, the roast pork sandwich, and, most famously of all, the cheesesteak. At Pat's and Geno's in South Philly you'll find the two most famous cheesesteak slingers in the city, fierce rivals positioned right across the street from each other. Philadelphians might want our heads, but the truth must be told: Neither is any good. The quality of meat is low, the seasoning is timid, and the cheese is a viscous Technicolor yellow goo (just because Cheez Whiz is traditional doesn't make it right). Our version uses tender, intensely beefy skirt steak, provolone, and a trio of caramelized vegetables to do the cheesesteak titans one better (for about 500 fewer calories).

You'll Need:

- 1 lb skirt or flank steak
- ½ Tbsp canola or peanut oil, plus more if needed
- 1 large yellow onion, diced
- 1 medium green bell pepper, diced
- 2 cups sliced mushrooms
- Salt and black pepper to taste
- 4 slices provolone
- 4 whole-wheat hoagie rolls, lightly toasted

How to Make It:

- Place the steak in the freezer for 20 minutes to firm up (this will help you slice it). Use a very sharp knife to cut the thinnest strips possible from the beef.

- Heat the oil in a large cast-iron skillet over medium heat. Add the onions and cook for about 5 minutes, until soft and lightly browned. Add the bell pepper and mushrooms and continue to cook for 5 to 7 minutes, until all of the vegetables are browned. Remove and reserve.

- Swirl in enough oil to coat the bottom of the pan and add the sliced steak. Season with salt and pepper right away, then use a spatula or tongs to keep the steak moving. After the steak has browned on all sides (because it's thin, this will happen quickly—4 to 5 minutes), stir in the reserved vegetables.

- Within the pan, divide the steak and veggie mixture into 4 equal piles and top each with a slice of provolone. Continue cooking for about 1 minute, just until the provolone has melted. Serve each pile on a hoagie roll.

Makes 4 servings

Per Serving
$3.93
540 calories
25 g fat
(10 g saturated)
790 mg sodium

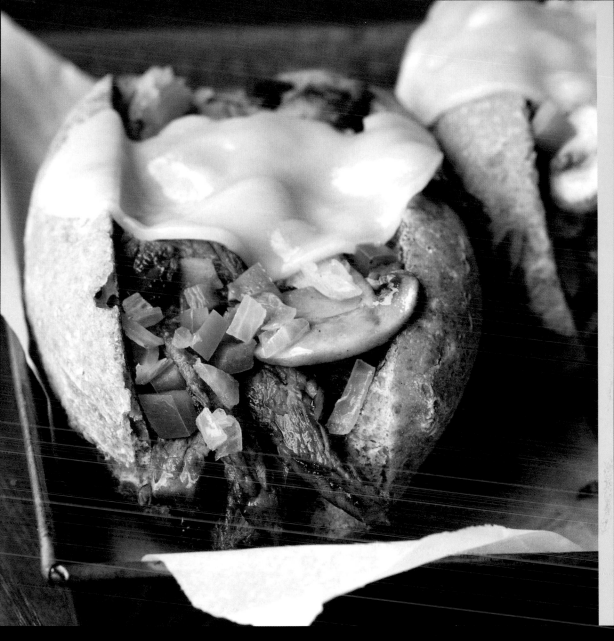

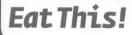

Buffalo Chicken & Blue Cheese Sandwich

Given the rate of wing consumption in this country, clearly hot sauce-slathered chicken and blue cheese is a winning combination for American palates. We stay true to the flavors people love—basting the chicken in hot sauce butter after grilling, topping with a yogurt-based blue cheese sauce—but manage to do what no one else out there has done yet: make Buffalo chicken into a healthy meal. Try the same technique with grilled shrimp.

You'll Need:

- ¼ cup crumbled blue cheese
- ½ cup Greek-style yogurt
- Juice of half a lemon
- Salt and pepper to taste
- 4 chicken breasts (6 oz each)
- ½ Tbsp chili powder
- 1 red onion, sliced
- 3 Tbsp favorite hot sauce (Frank's RedHot works best here)
- 2 Tbsp butter, melted in the microwave for 20 seconds
- 4 large romaine lettuce leaves
- 4 sesame seed buns, toasted

How to Make It:

- Preheat a grill or grill pan. While it's heating, combine the blue cheese, yogurt, and lemon juice, plus a pinch of salt and pepper. Stir to combine, and set aside.

- Season the chicken breasts with salt, pepper, and the chili powder. Add the chicken to the hot grill and cook for 4 to 5 minutes on the first side, then flip. Add the onions to the perimeter of the grill (if using a grill pan, you'll need to wait until you remove the chicken to grill the onions). Cook the chicken until firm and springy to the touch, another 4 to 5 minutes. Remove, along with the grilled onions.

- Combine the hot sauce and butter and brush all over the chicken after removing from the grill. Place one large leaf of romaine on the base of each bun. Top with a chicken breast, the blue cheese sauce, grilled onions, and then the top half of the bun.

Makes 4 servings

Per Serving
$3.81
387 calories
15 g fat
(5 g saturated)
912 mg sodium

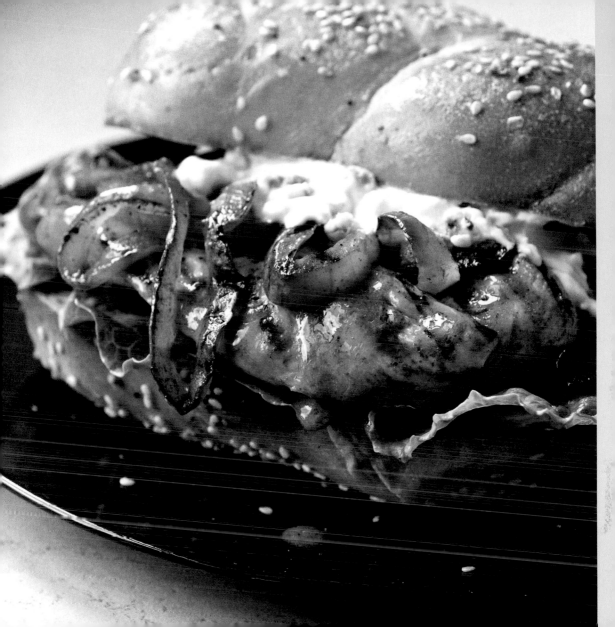

Eat This!

Ultimate Club Sandwich with Super Mayo

There are many people who believe that you can judge the quality of a hotel by its club sandwich. The reason being that it's the one item you will find on nearly all room service menus, and a place that puts love into the sandwich is likely putting love into the other small things that make a hotel great. We think our version—ham, turkey, bacon, and a souped-up mayo—would win over any guest, with the added bonus of containing half the calories of the club sandwiches that normally show up on the room service cart.

You'll Need:

- 2 Tbsp olive oil mayonnaise
- 1 Tbsp Dijon mustard
- 1 clove garlic, finely minced (or grated on a microplane)
- 1 tsp dried oregano
- 6 sandwich rolls, split and lightly toasted (12 pieces total; see Secret Weapon, right)
- 2 cups shredded romaine
- 8 slices tomato
- 8 strips cooked bacon
- 4 oz ham in 8 slices
- 4 oz turkey in 8 slices

How to Make It:

- In a mixing bowl combine the mayonnaise, mustard, garlic, and oregano.
- Spread the mayo mixture on 8 pieces of the toasted sandwich rolls. Top each piece with shredded romaine, a slice of tomato, and a strip of bacon. Top 4 of the pieces with ham and the other 4 with turkey.
- Build each sandwich with a turkey half, a ham half, and top with a final piece of sandwich roll for a tri-level sandwich.

Makes 4 servings

Per Serving

$2.68

330 calories
12 g fat
(2.5 g saturated)
980 mg sodium

SECRET WEAPON

Sandwich Thins

Most club sandwiches are more refined carbs than meat or produce—the extra layer of bread adding nothing but excess calories to the mix. Our version is built on sandwich rolls (aka sandwich thins), great low-calorie, high-fiber bread now widely available throughout North America. Both Oroweat and Nature's Own make varieties that contain just 100 calories and pack 5 grams of fiber per roll—more fiber and fewer calories than you'd get with two slices of whole-wheat bread. Make these your go-to sandwich vessels.

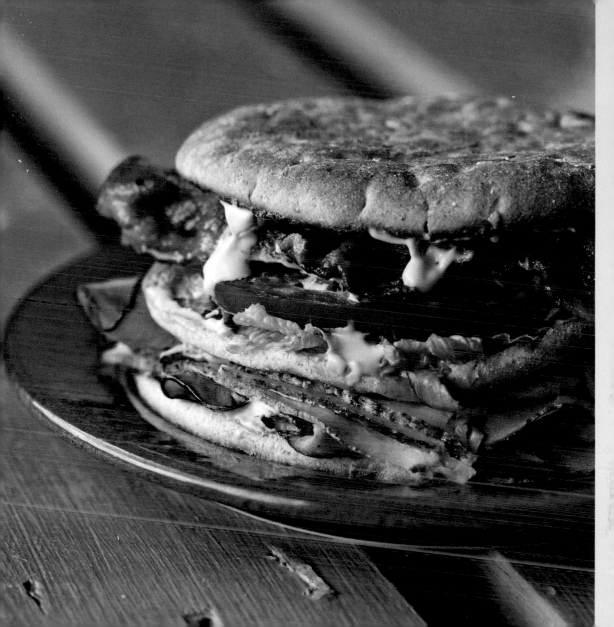

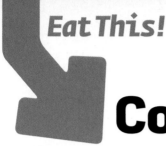

Eat This!

Cowboy Burger

We're not afraid to admit when a fast-food joint has a good idea. The inspiration for this burger comes from a Carl's Jr. classic, the Western Bacon Cheeseburger, a how-can-it-not-be-delicious commingling of beef, barbecue sauce, and fried onions. Problem is, the small version of Carl's burger packs 740 calories and a full day's worth of saturated fat. This version uses naturally lean bison and replaces the breaded onion rings with sweet grilled ones.

You'll Need:

- 1 lb ground bison or beef sirloin
- 1 medium red onion, sliced into ¼"-thick rings and skewered with toothpicks
- ½ Tbsp finely ground coffee
- 1 tsp chipotle or ancho chile powder
- Salt and black pepper to taste
- 4 slices sharp Cheddar
- 4 sesame seed buns, lightly toasted
- 6 strips bacon, cooked until crisp and halved
- 4 Tbsp Classic Barbecue Sauce (page 319 or store-bought)

We have no idea if cowboys actually eat burgers, but if they did, they would taste an awful lot like this one.

How to Make It:

- Gently form the beef into 4 patties, being careful not to overwork the meat. Let the patties rest for 15 minutes.

- Preheat the grill or grill pan over medium heat. Grill the onion slices, turning, for about 10 minutes, until soft and lightly charred. Just before cooking the patties, season them on both sides with the coffee, chile powder, and salt and pepper. Grill the patties alongside the onions for about 4 minutes, until nicely browned. Flip, top with the cheese, and continue grilling for 3 to 4 minutes longer, until the centers of the patties are firm but gently yielding to the touch and an instant-read thermometer inserted into the thickest part of a burger registers 135°F.

- Place the burgers on the bun bottoms, top with onions, bacon, and barbecue sauce.

Makes 4 servings

— *Normally we're not huge fans of heavily spiced burgers, but the coffee here adds a roasted depth to the burger that pairs beautifully with the barbecue sauce and bacon.*

Per Serving
$2.62
460 calories
22 g fat
(11 g saturated)
850 mg sodium

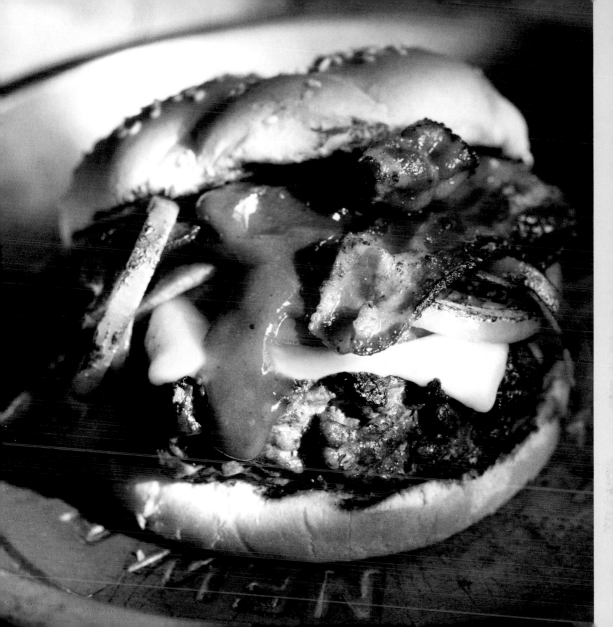

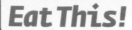

Roast Beef & Cheddar Sandwiches with Horseradish Mayo

The journey to sandwich enlightenment requires careful provisioning: fresh bread, high-quality produce, and the best meat you can get your hands on. Unfortunately, most prepackaged deli cuts are overloaded with sodium, nitrites, and other unsavory additives. We prefer to use leftover roasted or grilled meats—steak, chicken, pork chops—or failing that, buy meats from a supermarket deli department that does the roasting themselves. In the best possible world, the filling for this spicy sandwich would come from the Garlic-Rosemary Roast Beef on page 208.

You'll Need:

- 2 Tbsp olive oil mayonnaise
- 2 Tbsp Greek yogurt
- 2 Tbsp prepared horseradish
- 1 Tbsp Dijon mustard
- 1 clove garlic, finely minced
- 2 cups arugula
- 8 slices multigrain bread, lightly toasted
- 1 large tomato, sliced
- ½ red onion, very thinly sliced
- 1 lb leftover Garlic-Rosemary Roast Beef (page 208), thinly sliced, or high-quality store-bought roast beef
- 4 slices sharp Cheddar

How to Make It:

- Combine the mayo, yogurt, horseradish, Dijon, and garlic in a mixing bowl.
- Divide the arugula among 4 pieces of bread. Top with the tomato slices (seasoned with a pinch of salt), onion slices, roast beef, and Cheddar. Spread the top pieces of bread with a thick layer of the horseradish mayo and complete the sandwiches.

Makes 4 servings

Per Serving
$3.43
400 calories
20 g fat
(7 g saturated)
780 mg sodium

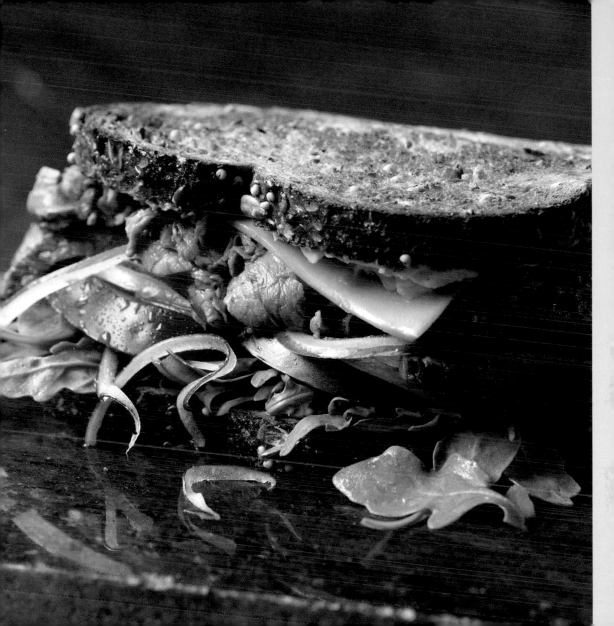

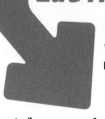

Eat This!

Southwest Turkey Burger

A few years back, Carl's Jr. and Hardee's reached out to us and asked for help designing a line of turkey burgers that would improve an otherwise high-calorie menu. A lot of time and testing went into the burgers, during which we learned just how well turkey takes to intense, vibrant flavors that might not jibe as well with beef. In the end, this spicy-cool burger didn't make it on the menu, but it remains one of the best turkey burgers we've had.

You'll Need:

- 2 Tbsp olive oil mayonnaise
- 1 Tbsp chipotle puree
- 1 Tbsp lime juice
- 1 lb ground turkey
- 1 Tbsp Magic Blackening Rub (page 320)

Salt and black pepper to taste

- 4 slices pepper Jack or Monterey Jack cheese
- 4 English muffins or potato rolls, lightly toasted
- 1 avocado, pitted, peeled, and thinly sliced
- ½ cup Pico de Gallo (page 319)

How to Make It:

- In a mixing bowl, combine the mayo, chipotle puree, and lime juice. Reserve.
- Preheat a grill, grill pan, or cast-iron skillet over medium heat. Gently form the turkey into 4 equal patties (being careful not to overwork the meat, which makes for dense, tough burgers). Season both sides of the burgers with the blackening rub, plus salt and black pepper.
- Cook the burgers on the grill for about 4 minutes, until a nice dark crust has formed on the bottoms. Flip and immediately cover with the cheese. Continue cooking for about 4 minutes longer, until the cheese is melted and the burger is just firm to the touch. Top 4 English muffin halves with the avocado slices and Pico de Gallo, then place a burger on top of each. Spoon the chipotle mayo over the burgers and serve.

Makes 4 servings.

MEAL MULTIPLIER

We tested dozens of creations for the Carl's Jr.–Hardee's turkey burger project. Here are three of the best outtakes that you can create at home.

- Grilled pineapple, Swiss cheese, teriyaki sauce
- Thinly sliced apple, Brie, honey mustard
- Ham, Swiss, spicy mustard, and pickles, toasted on the outside like a Cuban sandwich

Per Serving
$2.88
470 calories
26 g fat
(7 g saturated)
520 mg sodium

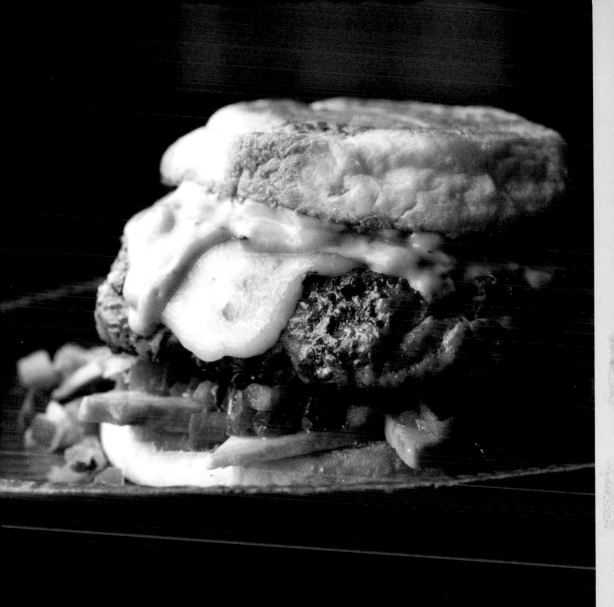

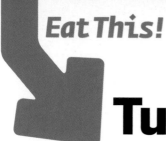

Turkey Sloppy Joe

It's amazing that multiple companies make a living selling packets, boxes, and cans of sloppy joe mix, many of them loaded with funky preservatives and fillers that even chemists would have a difficult time deciphering. All in the name of shaving 30 seconds from your total cooking time. The best part about sloppy joes is that everything you need is likely already in your pantry and spice cabinet, gathering dust, waiting for a chance to shine. Open a can, measure out a few spices (if you have children, employ them as your sous chefs), and you'll have a crowd-pleasing dinner on the table in about 15 minutes.

You'll Need:

½ Tbsp olive oil

1 large onion, diced

1 green bell pepper, diced

1 lb lean ground turkey

1½ cups tomato sauce

2 Tbsp tomato paste

2 Tbsp brown sugar

1 Tbsp red wine vinegar

1 Tbsp Worcestershire sauce

½ Tbsp chili powder

10–12 shakes Tabasco or other hot sauce

Salt and black pepper to taste

4 whole-wheat or sesame rolls, split and toasted

How to Make It:

● Heat the oil in a large skillet or sauté pan over medium heat. Add the onion and bell pepper and cook for about 2 minutes, until softened. Add the turkey and cook, using a wooden spoon to break up the meat, until the turkey is lightly browned. Add the tomato sauce, tomato paste, sugar, vinegar, Worcestershire, chili powder, and hot sauce and season with salt and pepper.

● Turn the heat down to low. Simmer for 10 minutes, until the liquid has reduced and the sauce fully coats the meat. Divide the mixture among the rolls.

Makes 4 servings

Lean ground sirloin or chicken works just as well here as turkey. As crazy as it sounds, so does a few fillets of finely chopped catfish—the perfect way to sneak fish into your family's diet.

Per Serving
$2.07
340 calories

11 g fat
(2.5 g saturated)

820 mg sodium

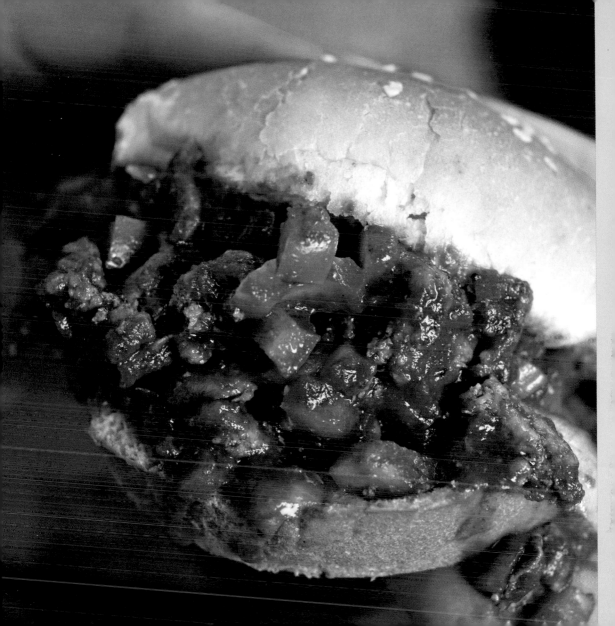

Eat This!

Swiss Burger with Red Wine Mushrooms

One of the many by-products of the Great Burger Boom of the 21st Century is what you might call the bourgie burger. You'll recognize it by its exotic condiments and its 20-syllable menu name. Even chains like Ruby Tuesday and Chili's have tried their hands at the bourgie burger—with predictably precarious results. Our take on the upscale burger is a snap to make, tastes like it costs 20 bucks, and packs fewer calories than an average salad.

You'll Need:

- 2 strips bacon, chopped
- 1 medium onion, sliced
- 1 clove garlic, minced
- 4 oz cremini mushrooms, sliced
- ½ cup red wine
- 2 Tbsp balsamic vinegar
- Salt and black pepper to taste
- 1 lb ground sirloin
- ½ cup shredded Gruyère or other Swiss cheese
- 2 cups arugula
- 4 potato buns, lightly toasted on the insides

How to Make It:

- Cook the bacon in a large sauté pan over medium heat for 5 minutes, until browned and crispy. Remove and reserve. Drain off all but a teaspoon of the bacon fat, then return the pan to the stove.
- Add the onions and garlic and cook for 5 minutes, until the onions are lightly browned. Add the mushrooms and continue cooking for 3 to 4 minutes, until the mushrooms are soft. Add the red wine and balsamic and simmer until the liquid begins to cling to the vegetables. Fold in the reserved bacon. Season with salt and black pepper.
- Preheat a grill, grill pan, or cast-iron skillet over medium heat. Gently form the sirloin into 4 equal patties. Season the patties on both sides with salt and pepper and cook for about 4 minutes, until nicely charred on the bottoms. Flip, immediately cover with the cheese, and continue cooking for another 4 minutes, until the cheese is melted and the burgers are firm but gently yielding to the touch.
- Place a handful of arugula on the bottom of each bun and top with a burger. Divide the mushroom mixture among the 4 burgers and top with the bun tops.

Makes 4 servings

Per Serving
$1.90
390 calories
13 g fat
(5 g saturated)
360 mg sodium

$$(\Psi + \mathsf{I})^2$$

MEAL MULTIPLIER

Other fancy-pants burger ideas:

- Lamb burgers with grilled eggplant, roasted peppers, feta cheese
- Tuna burgers with roasted red peppers, Chimichurri (page 319)
- Ground brisket burgers with smoked Cheddar and caramelized onions

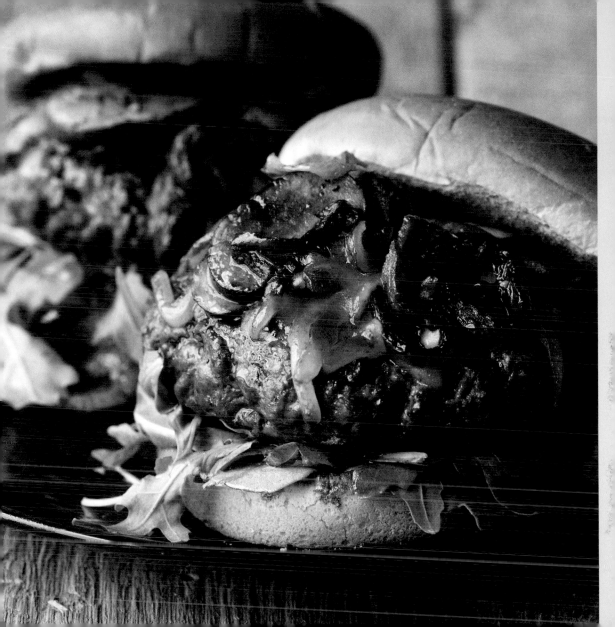

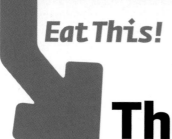

Eat This!

The Elvis

By now, most of us have heard the stories about Elvis's prodigious powers of consumption, and, in particular, his love of a certain sandwich involving peanut butter, banana, and, according to some accounts, bacon and honey. We take those accounts seriously, which is why, to honor the King, we bring them all together in this sandwich. But don't worry, this version is considerably more modest than most of Presley's creations (one, called the Fool's Gold Loaf, consisted of a hollowed-out loaf of bread stuffed with a pound of bacon and a jar each of peanut butter and grape jelly). The King isn't the only lover of this sweet and salty combination; New York City Mayor Michael Bloomberg once said that the Elvis would be his last meal.

You'll Need:

- ¼ cup smooth natural peanut butter
- 8 slices whole-wheat bread, lightly toasted
- 2 bananas, sliced
- 1 Tbsp honey
- 2 slices bacon, cooked and crumbled

You can add more bacon if you like, but we find a modest sprinkle gives the sandwich all the smoky, savory kick it needs.

How to Make It:

- Spread a generous layer of peanut butter on 4 pieces of the toast. Pave with the banana slices, drizzle with a light stream of honey, and scatter with the crumbled bacon pieces. Top with the remaining toast.

Makes 4 servings

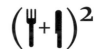

MEAL MULTIPLIER

Our last meal on this earth wouldn't be the Elvis, but another bacon-fueled sandwich phenom: the BLT. While it's nearly perfect on its own, these are a few modifications worth exploring:

- **BATE:** Bacon, Arugula, Tomato, and a sunny-side-up Egg
- **BLAT:** Bacon, Lettuce (preferably romaine), Avocado, and Tomato
- **BLATSM:** Bacon, Lettuce, Avocado, Tomato, Sriracha-spiked Mayo

Per Serving
$0.87
330 calories
12 g fat
(2.5 g saturated)
360 mg sodium

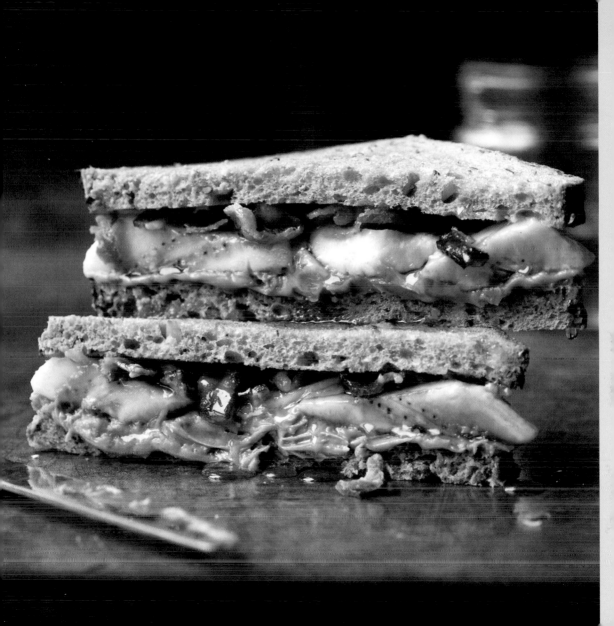

PIZZAS & PASTA

America's Worst PIZZAS & PASTAS

Domino's Deep Dish ExtravaganZZa Feast
(2 slices, large pie)

780 calories
36 g fat (14 g saturated)
1,940 mg sodium
**Price: $14.99
($3.75 for 2 slices)**

When did pizza get so complicated? A bit of cheese, a single source of protein, and a veggie or two was working just fine, but today's delivery menus are teeming with pies, like this one, that pull out all the heart-stopping stops—extra cheese, multiple meats, fancy crusts—at a high cost to your waistline and your wallet. Make pizza a comfort food you prepare in the comfort of your kitchen.

Eat This Instead!

Spicy Hawaiian Pizza
(page 152)

490 calories
24 g fat
(9 g saturated)
980 mg sodium
Cost per serving: $2.42
Save! 290 calories and $1.33!

146

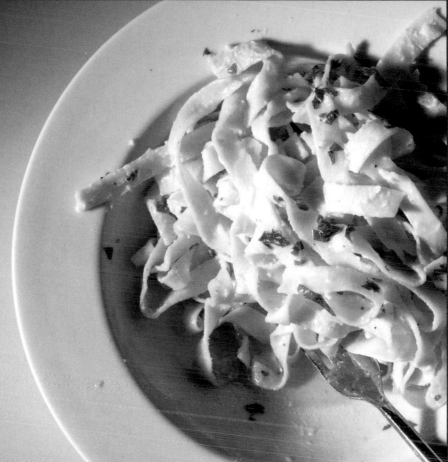

82 grams of saturated fat

Cheesecake Factory and fettuccine Alfredo: a diabolical partnership.

WORST LASAGNA
Olive Garden's Lasagna Rollata al Forno

1,170 calories
68 g fat (39 g saturated)
2,510 mg sodium
Price: $13.95

Having trouble deciphering the long Italian name? Here, we'll translate for you: handkerchiefs of pasta stuffed with five types of cheese, topped with more cheese, covered in a sauce also made with five cheeses, then baked until all that pasta and cheese dissolves into a soup of saturated fat. Olive Garden likes to market itself as an outpost of some fantasy Tuscan restaurant, but if any Italian saw this plate, he'd book the first flight back to the motherland.

Eat This Instead!
Sausage Lasagna
(page 164)

360 calories
11 g fat (5 g saturated)
450 mg sodium
Cost per serving: $1.69
Save! 810 calories and $12.26!

WORST PERSONAL PIZZA
Uno Chicago Grill's Individual Chicago Classic Deep Dish Pizza

2,240 calories
156 g fat (48 g saturated)
4,4400 mg sodium
Price: $10.59

Where to begin? With the fact that this pie has more calories than four Big Macs?

How about the eye-popping saturated fat number—equivalent to 53 slices of Hormel Center Cut Bacon? Let's not forget the sodium, a number so astronomical that it haunts cardiologists the country over. But the most appalling part about this pizza—our pick for the Worst Pizza in America for five years running—is that Uno's has the audacity to call it an "individual" pie.

Eat This Instead!
Spinach, Sausage & Pepper Pizza (page 158)

460 calories
20 g fat (8 g saturated)
780 mg sodium
Cost per serving: $2.79
Save! 1,780 calories and $7.80!

WORST MACARONI AND CHEESE
Uno Chicago Grill's Macaroni and Cheese

1,860 calories
107 g fat (53 g saturated)
2,860 mg sodium
Price: $12.49

When it comes to comfort foods, mac and cheese is numero uno. When it comes to dietary discomfort, Uno Chicago takes the cheese. Alright, cheesy puns aside, there's nothing comforting about taking in a day's worth of calories and 3 days' worth of saturated fat in one sitting. Mac and cheese can be done right—or at least done reasonable—but it takes quality ingredients and

tame portions, two scarce resources in the land of American chains.

Eat This Instead!
Mac and Cheese (page 150)

360 calories
16 g fat (8 g saturated)
560 mg sodium
Cost per serving: $1.28
Save! 1,500 calories and $11.21!

WORST FETTUCCINE ALFREDO
Cheesecake Factory's Fettuccini Alfredo

1,830 calories
N/A g fat (82 g saturated)
1,071 mg sodium
Price: $14.50

Considering that Alfredo is consistently the worst Italian-American offering on any chain menu, and that the Cheesecake Factory is consistently the worst chain restaurant in America, we can't say we were shocked to discover that this noodle plate packs more than 5 days' worth of saturated fat. We are surprised that people continue to pay good money for such a dangerous dish when a better, cheaper, healthier version can be made in minutes at home.

Eat This Instead!
Fettuccine Alfredo
(page 156)

460 calories
11 g fat (6 g saturated)
480 mg sodium
Cost per serving: $1.18
Save! 1,370 calories and $13.32!

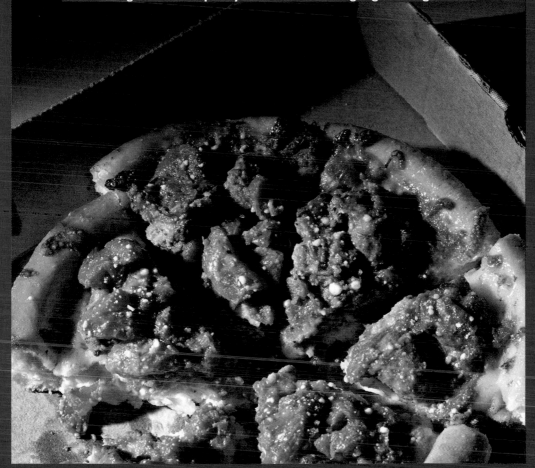

1,860 calories

Uno's Chicago Classic: the pizza you want to eat before going on a hunger strike.

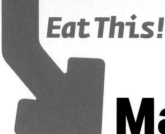

Mac & Cheese

Mac and cheese: the undisputed king of comfort food. Over the years, we've tested dozens of iterations of the classic—spiked with chiles, goosed with bacon, toned down with nonfat cheese. But we keep returning to this formula: a béchamel base, laced with extra-sharp Cheddar cheese, and finished with a bit of yogurt to give the sauce that perfect texture. Are there more decadent bowls of mac? Absolutely, but not for under 400 calories.

You'll Need:

- 2 cups elbow macaroni, fusilli, or cavatappi pasta
- 2 Tbsp butter
- 2 Tbsp flour
- 2 cups 2% milk
- 1½ cups shredded extra sharp Cheddar
- ½ cup grated Parmesan
- ¼ cup Greek yogurt
- ½ cup panko bread crumbs
- Black pepper to taste

Real Italian Parmesan is called Parmigiano-Reggiano and its sharp, nutty flavor has nothing in common with the stuff you shake from a green can. It may be a bit pricey, but a little goes a long way.

How to Make It:

- Cook the pasta according to package directions until just al dente. Drain and reserve.

- While the pasta cooks, melt the butter in a medium saucepan over medium heat. Stir in the flour and cook, stirring, for 1 minute. Slowly add the milk, whisking to prevent lumps from forming. Simmer the béchamel for 5 minutes, until it begins to thicken to the consistency of heavy cream. Stir in the Cheddar and ¼ cup of the Parmesan and cook until completely melted. Cut the heat and stir in the yogurt. Add the pasta and toss to evenly coat.

- Preheat the broiler. Pour the macaroni and cheese into an 8" x 8" baking dish (or into individual ramekins). Top with the bread crumbs and the remaining Parmesan and season with black pepper. Place on the middle rack of the oven and broil for 5 to 7 minutes, until the bread crumbs are golden brown.

Makes 4 servings

Per Serving
$1.28
360 calories
16 g fat
(8 g saturated)
560 mg sodium

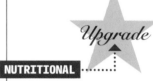

Upgrade

NUTRITIONAL

Yes, this mac and cheese is fantastically low in calories when compared with restaurant and frozen versions out there, but that being said, there is always room for improvement. Cut calories by swapping in low-fat cheese for the full-fat Cheddar; add fiber by using whole-wheat or fortified pasta (preferably Ronzoni Smart Taste) instead of white noodles; and boost nutrition by stirring in steamed broccoli, cherry tomatoes, roasted peppers, even a few scoops of salsa.

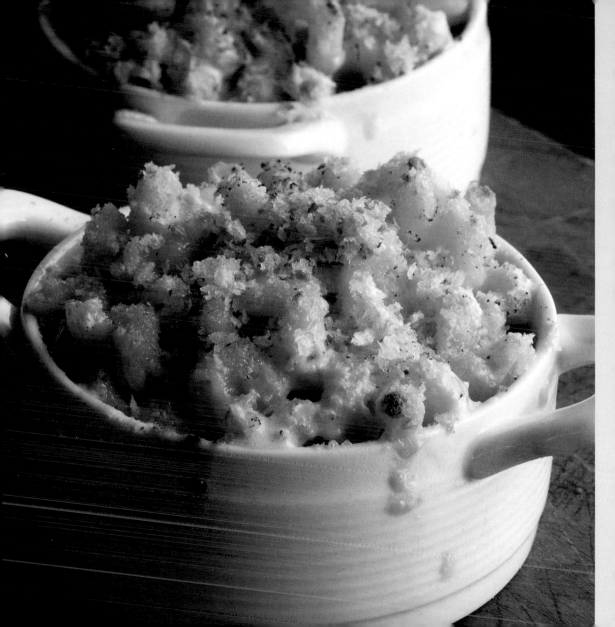

Spicy Hawaiian Pizza

Specialty pies are the bane of the pizza world. Look at any nutritional guide from the major pizza purveyors and you'll see calories, fat, and sodium jump dramatically as you move from simple pizzas to the elaborate concoctions the pizza execs dream up. (Do you really need pepperoni, sausage, bacon, *and* ground beef on your pie?) When it comes to funky pies, though, we've long had a love affair with the Hawaiian, not just for its yin-yang balance of sweetness and smoke, but also because it's one of the healthiest pizzas you can eat. It might not be authentic Italian, but it's authentically American.

You'll Need:

1 package instant yeast

1 cup hot water

½ tsp salt

1 Tbsp honey

½ Tbsp olive oil

2½ cups flour, plus more for kneading and rolling (or 2 thin-crust store-bought pizza shells)

1 cup Tomato Sauce (page 321)

1 cup diced fresh mozzarella (or 1 cup shredded low-moisture mozzarella)

1 cup chopped pineapple

4 slices smoked ham (like Black Forest), cut into chunks

1 small red onion, thinly sliced

1 jalapeño pepper, thinly sliced

How to Make It:

- Combine the yeast with the water, salt, and honey. Allow to sit for 10 minutes while the hot water activates the yeast. Stir in the olive oil and flour, using a wooden spoon to incorporate. When the dough is no longer sticky, place on a cutting board, cover with more flour, and knead for 5 minutes. Return to the bowl, cover with plastic wrap, and let the dough rise at room temperature for at least 90 minutes.

- Preheat the oven to 500°F. If you have a pizza stone, place it on the bottom rack of the oven.

- On a lightly floured surface, stretch the dough into two 12" circles. Working with one pizza at a time, place the pizza shell on a baking sheet, cover with a thin layer of tomato sauce, then top with half of the cheese, pineapple, ham, onion, and jalapeño. (If using a pizza stone, do this on a floured pizza peel, then slide the pizza onto the stone for baking.) Bake for about 8 minutes, until the cheese is melted and bubbling and the crust is golden brown. Repeat to make the second pizza. Cut each pie into 6 slices.

Makes 4 servings

Per Serving
$2.42
490 calories
24 g fat
(9 g saturated)
980 mg sodium

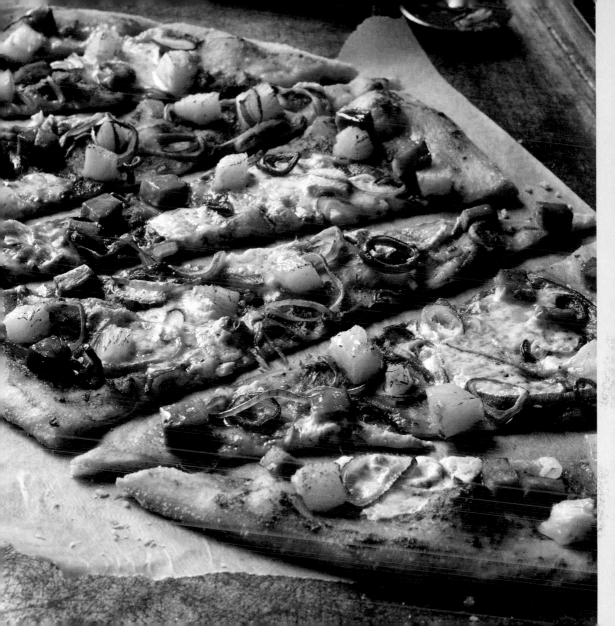

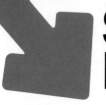

Spinach-Artichoke Manicotti with Spicy Tomato Sauce

There are a thousand ways to stuff a piece of pasta—from three-cheese ravioli to a meaty, saucy tower of lasagna—but the one common denominator is a deluge of calories and an abundance of sodium. To deliver the creature comforts of red-sauce Italian food, we keep the cheesy stuffing, but to make it something you can feel good about eating, we use low-fat ricotta and cottage cheese cut with plenty of sautéed spinach and artichoke hearts.

You'll Need:

- 1 Tbsp olive oil
- 3 cloves garlic, minced
- 1 jar (6 oz) marinated artichoke hearts
- 1 bag (10 oz) frozen spinach, thawed
- Salt and black pepper to taste
- 1 small onion, minced
- ½ tsp red pepper flakes
- 1 can (28 oz) crushed tomatoes
- 12 manicotti tubes
- ½ cup low-fat ricotta cheese
- ¼ cup low-fat cottage cheese
- ¼ cup grated Parmesan
- ½ cup shredded mozzarella

How to Make It:

- Preheat the oven to 350°F.
- Heat half the olive oil in a medium sauté pan over medium heat. Add one-third of the garlic and sauté for about 1 minute, until soft and light brown. Add the artichoke hearts and spinach. Cook for about 3 minutes, until the vegetables are warmed through. Drain any water that collects in the bottom of the pan. Season with salt and black pepper.
- Heat the remaining olive oil in a medium saucepan over medium heat. Add the remaining garlic, the onions, and red pepper flakes and cook for about 3 minutes, until the onion is soft. Add the tomatoes and simmer for 10 minutes. Season with salt and pepper.
- While the sauce simmers, cook the manicotti in a large pot of boiling water for about 7 minutes, until soft but short of al dente. Drain.
- Combine the artichoke-spinach mixture with the ricotta, cottage cheese, and Parmesan. Use a small spoon to carefully stuff each manicotti with the cheese mixture.
- Spoon half of the tomato sauce on the bottom of a 13" x 9" baking dish. Top with the manicotti, then cover with the remaining sauce. Sprinkle the mozzarella all over. Bake for about 20 minutes, until the cheese is melted and the sauce is bubbling.

Makes 4 servings

Per Serving
$2.63
450 calories
11 g fat
(4 g saturated)
810 mg sodium

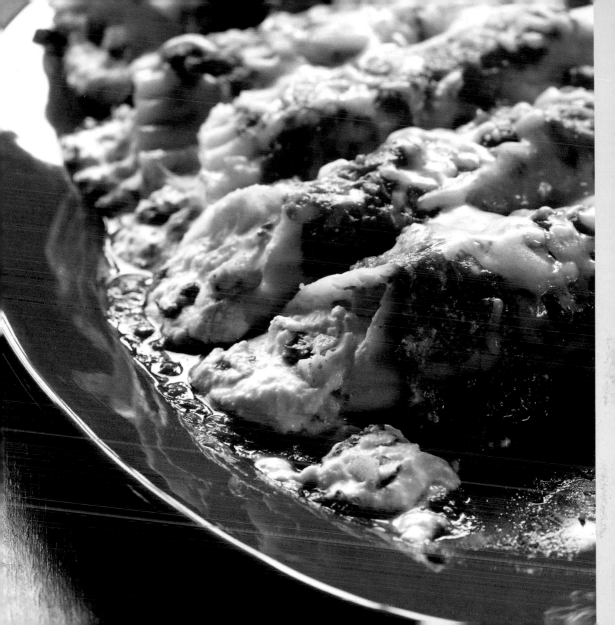

Fettuccine Alfredo

Alfredo di Lelio invented this iconic dish at his trattoria in Rome in 1914. Back then, the dish was nothing more than hot fettuccine tossed with butter and Parmesan cheese. Eventually fettuccine Alfredo made its way across the Atlantic, picking up a sea of heavy cream along the way. Now it's a staple on chain restaurant menus everywhere, not least of all because it costs next to nothing to load a bowl with 1,200 calories' worth of fat and refined carbohydrates. To dampen the Alfredo impact, we turn to our old friend béchamel, which creates a thick, creamy sauce without the calories of heavy cream and excess butter.

You'll Need:

1½ Tbsp butter

1 Tbsp flour

1½ cups low-fat milk

2 Tbsp Neufchâtel

½ cup grated Parmesan, plus more for serving

1 tsp grated lemon zest

Salt to taste

1 package (12 oz) fresh fettuccine

This low-cal cream cheese gives this sauce that perfect Alfredo creaminess.

How to Make It:

- Melt the butter in a medium saucepan over medium heat. Stir in the flour and cook, stirring, until golden brown. Add the milk, whisking to prevent any lumps from forming. Simmer for 5 minutes, until the sauce thickens. Stir in the Neufchâtel, Parmesan, lemon zest, and salt. Keep warm.

- While the sauce simmers, cook the pasta according to package instructions (remember, fresh pasta cooks in a fraction of the time it takes to cook dried pasta). Drain and add directly to the saucepan. Toss until the pasta is thoroughly coated, then divide among 4 warm pasta bowls. Serve with more grated Parmesan, if you like.

Makes 4 servings

Per Serving

$1.18

460 calories

11 g fat
(6 g saturated)

480 mg sodium

Upgrade

NUTRITIONAL

Alfredo isn't plagued by just the punishing calorie count, but also by the fact that it offers little in the way of protein, fiber, or anything resembling real nutrition. That's why we like to supplement our bowl with as many healthy add-ons as possible. Starting with this recipe as the base, add any combination of the following to the sauce just before tossing with the pasta: grilled chicken or shrimp, steamed broccoli, sautéed mushrooms, sautéed spinach, roasted asparagus, cherry tomatoes.

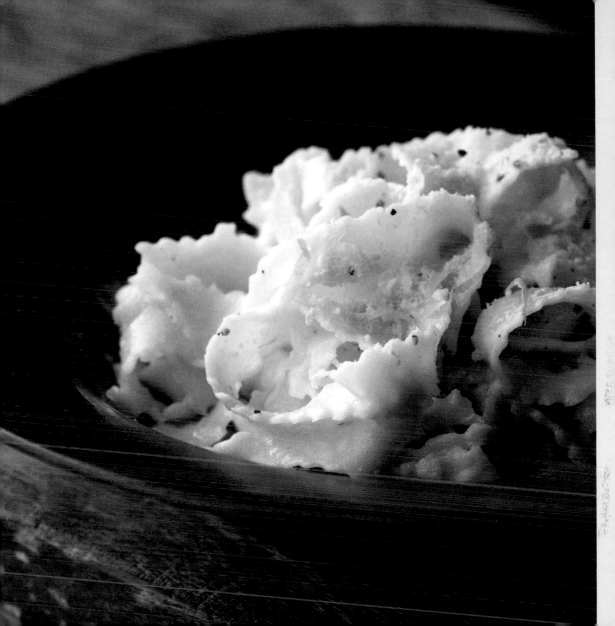

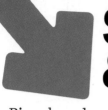

Eat This!

Spinach, Sausage & Pepper Pizza

Pizza has always been something people are happy to let someone else make for them—whether it's Domino's or DiGiorno or Dom, your local pizza dude. But industrially made pizza can not only be disappointing, but also really bad for you. Making pizza at home gives you ultimate quality control—over the freshness of the ingredients, the bulk of the crust, the combination of flavors. With a bit of practice, you'll outgun the best pizzerias in your town.

You'll Need:

- 1 tsp olive oil
- 2 links Italian-style chicken sausage, casings removed
- 1 clove garlic, minced
- 1 bunch spinach, cleaned and stemmed
- Salt and black pepper to taste
- Pizza Dough (page 152), or 2 thin-crust store-bought pizza shells
- 1 cup Tomato Sauce (page 321)
- 1 cup diced fresh mozzarella (or 1 cup shredded low-moisture mozzarella)
- ½ cup Peppadew peppers, or other bottled roasted peppers

How to Make It:

- Preheat the oven to 500°F. If you have a pizza stone, place it on the bottom rack of the oven.

- Heat the olive oil in a large pan over medium heat. Add the sausage and cook for about 3 minutes, until no longer pink. Add the garlic and cook for 2 minutes more. Add the spinach and cook, stirring, until wilted. Drain any excess liquid gathered at the bottom pan. Season with salt and pepper.

- On a lightly floured surface, stretch the dough into two 12" circles. Working with one pizza at a time, place the pizza shell on a baking sheet, cover with a thin layer of tomato sauce, then top with half the mozzarella, spinach-sausage mixture, and peppers. (If using a stone, do this on a floured pizza peel, then slide the pizza onto the stone for baking.) Bake for about 8 minutes, until the cheese is melted and bubbling and the crust is golden brown. Cut each pie into 6 pieces. Repeat to make the second pizza.

Makes 4 servings

Per Serving
$2.79
460 calories
20 g fat
(8 g saturated)
780 mg sodium

SECRET WEAPON

Peppadew Peppers

These tiny cherry-red peppers from South Africa pack an incredible one-two punch ozf sweet and heat, which makes them a wonderful addition to pizza, salads, pasta, and sandwiches. Or make a portable snack by stuffing them with pieces of fresh mozzarella or goat cheese. They're available by the jar in fancy supermarkets like Whole Foods, and often found sold by the pound in supermarket salad and olive bars. Still can't find them? Order jars online on amazon.com.

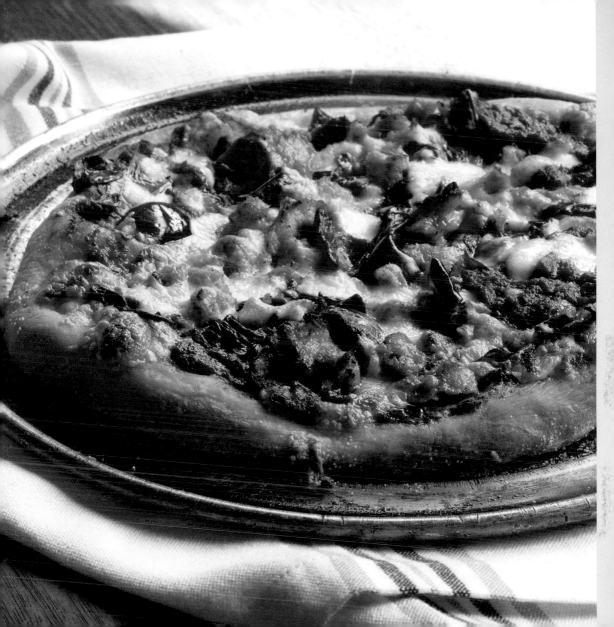

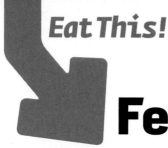

Fettuccine with Turkey Bolognese

Before there was spaghetti and meatballs, before there was tomato sauce with ground beef and Italian seasonings, before there was Hamburger Helper and bottles of Prego, there was ragù, a slow-simmered meat sauce that is heartier, more complex, and, yes, more comforting than its American counterparts.

You'll Need:

- ½ Tbsp olive oil
- 1 small onion, diced
- 2 stalks celery, diced
- 1 medium carrot, peeled and diced
- 2 cloves garlic, minced
- 8 oz ground white turkey
- 8 oz ground sirloin
- 1 link Italian-style turkey sausage, casing removed
- 1 cup dry white wine
- ½ cup 2% milk
- ½ cup low-sodium chicken stock
- 1 can (28 oz) crushed tomatoes
- 2 Tbsp tomato paste
- 1 bay leaf
- Salt and black pepper to taste
- 1 package (12 oz) fresh fettuccine or 8 oz dried egg noodles
- Finely grated Parmesan for serving

How to Make It:

- Heat the olive oil in a large saucepan over medium heat. Add the onion, celery, carrot, and garlic and sauté for 5 minutes, until softened. Add the ground turkey, sirloin, and sausage, using a wooden spoon to break the meat into small pieces. Cook for about 7 minutes, just until the meat is cooked through. Add the wine, milk, stock, tomatoes, tomato paste, and bay leaf. Turn the heat down to low and allow the sauce to simmer for at least 45 minutes (but preferably for up to 90 minutes over a very low flame). Season to taste with salt and pepper. Discard the bay leaf.

- Cook the pasta in salted boiling water until just al dente (usually 3 to 4 minutes with fresh pasta). Drain and return to the pot. Place on the stove over very low heat and add the Bolognese, a few big spoonfuls at a time, stirring so the sauce coats the noodles evenly. You will have more sauce than you need for the pasta (plan to use about two-thirds of what you've made). Divide the pasta among 4 warm bowls or plates. Pass the Parmesan at the table.

Makes 4 servings

Per Serving
$2.94
520 calories
10 g fat
(2.5 g saturated)
520 mg sodium

LEFTOVER♥LOVE

The Bolognese recipe makes more sauce than you need for this recipe (which is the point, since it only gets better the next day). Here are a few ways to repurpose the leftovers.

- Serve over soft polenta.
- Make a serious lasagna by layering no-bake noodles with béchamel, Parmesan, and the turkey Bolognese.
- Pile in a toasted bun like an Italian sloppy joe.

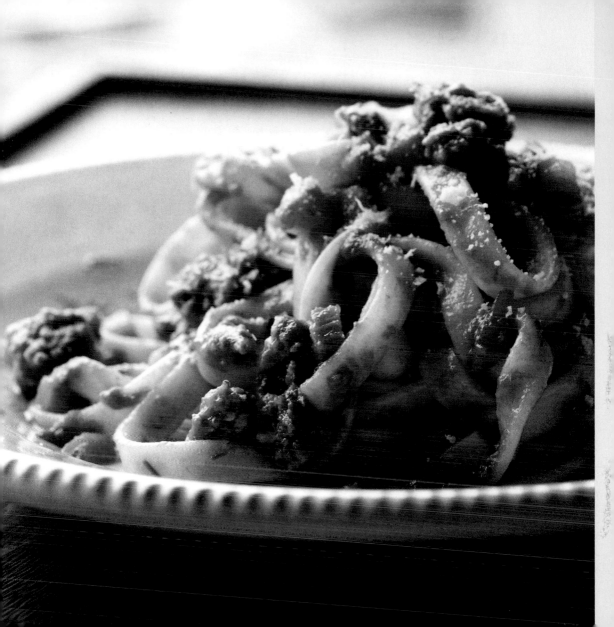

Spinach-&-Ham Mac & Cheese

This isn't your grandmama's mac and cheese. By introducing ham, spinach, and cherry tomatoes, we give the classic the nutritional juice it's never had before. More than just a health boost, though, the additions bring a level of nuance to a traditionally one-note (cheese!) dish. Improvise how you see fit (swap in broccoli for the spinach, turkey for the ham, Jack for the Swiss), but the core idea is one that will make mac and cheese a sustainable dinner staple.

You'll Need:

- 2 cups Ronzoni Smart Taste penne or whole-wheat penne
- 2 Tbsp butter
- 2 Tbsp flour
- 2 cups 2% milk
- Pinch of nutmeg
- 1 cup shredded fresh or 2% low-moisture mozzarella
- ½ cup shredded Swiss cheese
- ½ cup shredded Cheddar
- 4 oz smoked ham, chopped
- 1 cup steamed or sautéed spinach
- 1 cup cherry tomatoes, halved
- ½ cup panko bread crumbs
- Black pepper to taste

How to Make It:

- Cook the pasta according to package directions until just al dente. Drain and reserve.
- While the pasta cooks, melt the butter in a medium saucepan over medium heat. Stir in the flour and cook, stirring, for 1 minute to help eliminate the raw flour taste. Slowly add the milk, whisking to prevent lumps from forming. Simmer the béchamel for 5 minutes, until it begins to thicken to the consistency of heavy cream. Add the nutmeg and the cheeses and cook until fully melted. Add the pasta to the béchamel, along with the ham, spinach, and cherry tomatoes. Toss to distribute evenly.
- Preheat the broiler. Pour the macaroni and cheese into an 8" x 8" baking dish (or into individual ramekins). Top with the bread crumbs and season with black pepper. Place on the middle rack of the oven and broil for 5 to 7 minutes, until the bread crumbs are golden brown.

Makes 6 servings

Per Serving
$1.76
392 calories
15 g fat
(8 g saturated)
540 mg sodium

SECRET WEAPON

Ronzoni Smart Taste

We've tested most of the whole-wheat pastas on the market and we'd be lying if we didn't say that they left something to be desired. Perhaps that's being too generous; most have the texture and taste of wet cardboard coated in sand. That's why we love this line from Ronzoni. Smart Taste, a fortified white noodle, fuses the fiber of the best whole-wheat noodles with the smooth, toothsome texture of normal pasta. We recommend it for every pasta dish in this book, but it's especially vital in this manipulated mac.

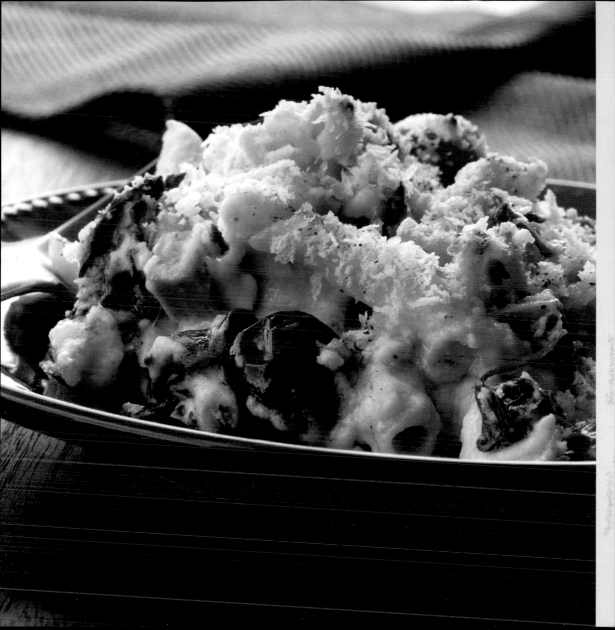

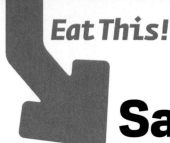

Eat This!

Sausage Lasagna

There are two types of lasagna in this world. The Italian type is made with a rich meat sauce and covered with béchamel instead of cheese, and the American type is heavy on tomatoes, ricotta, and mozzarella—a delicious, if not altogether healthy, interpretation. This version represents the best of both worlds, blending the cheesy, tomatoey comfort of the American version with the meatiness and relative healthfulness of the Italian take.

You'll Need:

- 1 Tbsp olive oil
- 3 links raw chicken sausage, casings removed
- 1 small onion, diced
- 2 cloves garlic, minced

Pinch red pepper flakes

- 1 can (28 oz) crushed tomatoes

Salt and black pepper to taste

- 1½ cups low-fat ricotta
- ½ cup 2% milk
- 16 sheets no-boil lasagna noodles •
- 16–20 fresh basil leaves
- 1 cup chopped fresh mozzarella

Barilla makes a good no-boil lasagna that is widely available.

How to Make It:

- Heat the olive oil in a large saucepan over medium heat. Add the sausage and cook for about 3 minutes, until no longer pink. Add the onion, garlic, and red pepper flakes and continue cooking for about 5 minutes, until the onion is soft and translucent. Add the tomatoes and simmer for 15 minutes. Season with salt and pepper.

- Preheat the oven to 350°F. Combine the ricotta and milk in a mixing bowl. In a 9" x 9" baking pan, lay down a layer of 4 noodles. Cover with a quarter of the ricotta mixture and a quarter of the sausage mixture, then a few basil leaves and a quarter of the mozzarella. Repeat three times to create a four-layer lasagna.

- Cover with aluminum foil and bake for 25 minutes, until the cheese is melted and the pasta cooked through. Remove the foil and increase the temperature to 450°F. Continue baking for about 10 minutes, until the top of the lasagna is nicely browned.

Makes 8 servings

Per Serving
$1.69
360 calories
11 g fat
(5 g saturated)
450 mg sodium

MEAL MULTIPLIER

Other ways to layer your lasagna:

- Sautéed mushrooms (as many different types as you can find), béchamel, and goat cheese
- Turkey Bolognese (page 160) and béchamel with a bit of grated Parmesan
- Shrimp sautéed with garlic and spinach, sun-dried tomatoes, and béchamel

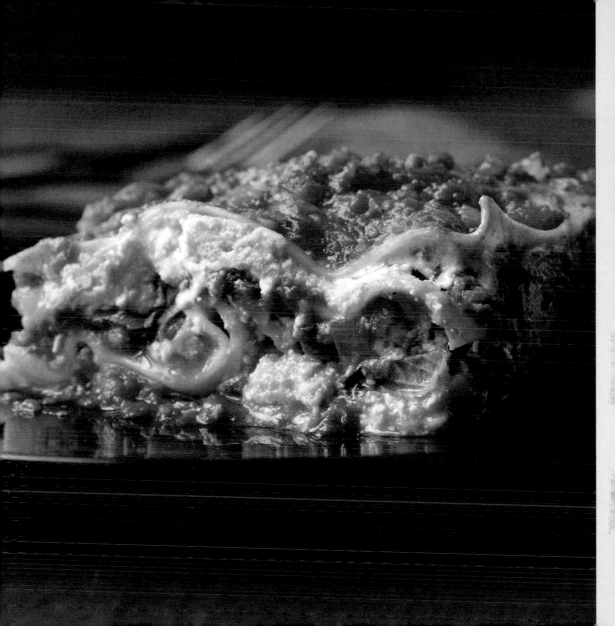

CHAPTER 7

POULTRY

America's Worst POULTRY

WORST CHICKEN PARMESAN
Applebee's Classic Chicken Parm

1,430 calories
58 g fat
(18 g saturated, 1 g trans)
3,140 mg sodium
Price: $11.49

"Parmesan." On its own, it's a simple word for an extraordinary Italian cheese. Attach it to beef, chicken, or even veggies (we're looking at you, eggplant!), and it becomes code for an oil-soaked, cheese-smothered Italian-American calorie bomb.

What's worse, the standard side dish for chicken parm at most chains
is a pile of refined pasta carbs. Luckily we've figured out a no-fuss baked version you can make at home that slashes calories and cost dramatically.

Eat This Instead!
Chicken Parm (page 188)

340 calories
9 g fat
(3.5 g saturated)
540 mg sodium
Cost per serving: $3.13
Save! 1,090 calories and $8.36!

WORST FRIED CHICKEN
Applebee's Chicken Fried Chicken

1,180 calories
60 g fat
(16 g saturated, 0.5 g trans)
2,780mg sodium
Price: $11.29

Nothing says down-home comfort like fried chicken, and while it's certainly not the most nutritious way to prepare your poultry, a modest serving of breaded bird won't kill you. But this Applebee's plate, with nearly a day's worth of trans fats and more sodium

168

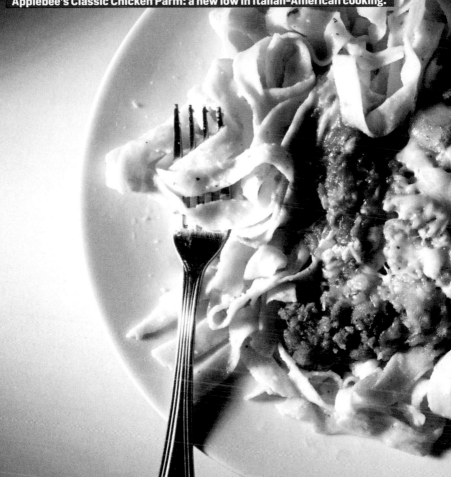

1,430 calories
Applebee's Classic Chicken Parm: a new low in Italian-American cooking.

than 21 small bags of Lay's potato chips, doesn't qualify as modest. We're big proponents of lean protein, but here, giant slabs of chicken breast just mean more surface area for grease-soaked breading. Toss in a smothering of country gravy that would make Paula Deen blush, and you have yourself some of the worst fried chicken in the United States.

Eat This Instead!
Oven-Fried Chicken
(page 184)

250 calories
14 g fat
(3 g saturated)
620 mg sodium
Cost per serving: $1.89
Save! 930 calories and $9.40!

WORST POTPIE
Perkins's Chicken Pot Pie

1,390 calories
102 g fat
(36 g saturated)
2,340 mg sodium
Price: $9.99

There are two surefire ways to ruin a perfectly lean piece of chicken: 1. Coat it in white flour and dunk it in the deep fryer. 2. Drown it in cream sauce and imprison it in a colossal cage of buttery quick-burning carbs. Potpie—stuffed with veggies and lean protein—can make for a hearty, heartening meal, but too often restaurants rely on cheap oils and massive portions, which guarantee that their poultry pots will supply you with a pot belly. And with as many calories as 30 McDonald's Chicken McNuggets, this Perkins pastry is the worst pot in the lot.

Eat This Instead!
Chicken Potpie (page 190)

350 calories
15 g fat
(8 g saturated)
650 mg sodium
Cost per serving: $3.84
Save! 1,040 calories and $6.15!

WORST ROASTED CHICKEN
Romano's Macaroni Grill's Chicken Under a Brick

1,590 calories
145 g fat
(31 g saturated)
2,040 mg sodium
Price: $16.00

The poor chicken never saw it coming—and we're not talking about the brick. The Tuscan grilling method of clobbering your poultry with a slab of clay can deliver lean, juicy meat, but Romano's gives its bird a double beating by drowning it in oil and salt—a maniacal maneuver that results in a dish with 75 percent of your daily calories and one and half days' worth of sodium. Stats like that will hit your waistline and blood pressure like a ton of, well, bricks.

Eat This Instead!
Sunday Roast Chicken
(page 176)

520 calories
27 g fat (7 g saturated)
820 mg sodium
Cost per serving: $3.07
Save! 1,070 calories and $12.93!

WORST CHICKEN
Cheesecake Factory's Crispy Chicken Costoletta

2,550 calories
N/A g fat (86 g saturated)
2,627 mg sodium
Price: $16.95

A "lightly breaded chicken breast" served with lemon sauce and fresh asparagus sounds like it could be the latest entrée from Lean Cuisine. Instead, it's a cautionary tale for people who think it's easy to spot the healthiest food on a restaurant menu. A diner chosing this chicken thinking it the lesser of the many Cheesecake Factory nutritional evils would be shocked to learn he would have been better off ordering three Factory Burgers than eating this combination.

Eat This Instead!
Provençal Chicken
(page 178)

340 calories
15 g fat
(2.5 g saturated)
680 mg sodium
Cost per serving: $2.77
Save! 2,210 calories and $14.18!

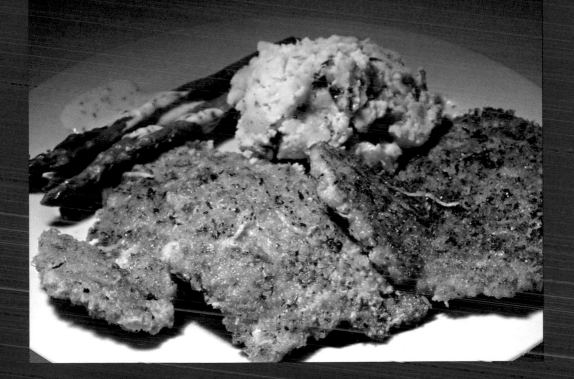

2,550 calories

In the bizzaro world that is the Cheesecake Factory, chicken, potatoes, and asparagus become one of the worst meals in America.

Slow Cooker

For most of us, time is a difficult element to corral. After sleep and work, our hours are few. Then there are dogs to walk, babies to change, and Kardashians to keep up with. When mealtime comes around, we favor convenience over substance—drive-thrus and frozen dinners over the fresh food we all want to eat after a long day.

So here's the million-dollar flat-belly question: Do skinny people have more time to eat healthfully? The answer: absolutely not. They have exactly the same number of minutes as you do. Their secret is in how they use those minutes.

The slow cooker is by no means the only way to eat better with less time,

but it is the most reliable. It's the only appliance that cooks for you—safely—while you're at work or in bed. It's more cost-effective than an oven, and unlike a stockpot on the stove, you don't have to worry about it boiling over or drying out your food. It's the kitchen alchemist, providing the slow, steady heat necessary to convert an onion's harsh volatiles into buttery sugars, soften hard winter beans into al dente starches, and transform tough, inexpensive cuts of meat into rich delicacies that fall apart with the softest pressure from your fork.

Yes, with the slow cooker on your side, a soul-warming comfort meal is as simple as a push of a button.

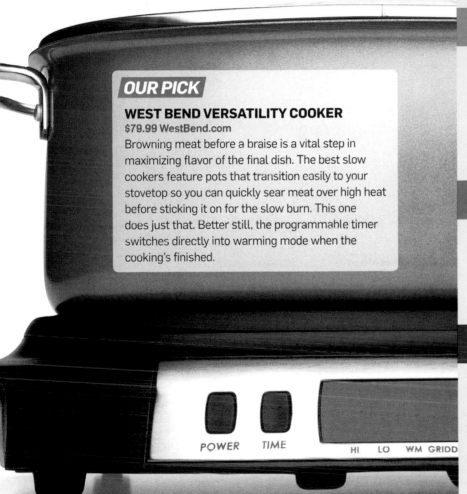

Slow-Cooker
SUPERPOWERS

TRANSFORM TOUGH CUTS

Combine big chunks of meat like sirloin, brisket, pork shoulder, or bone-in chicken with vegetables (onions, carrots), aromatics (garlic, herbs, spices), and a few cups of liquid (wine, stock, water, or beer). Set it and forget it. By the time you return, the meat will be perfectly tender and most of the fat will be left behind with the cooking liquid.

MAKE IT MEXICAN NIGHT

Combine chunks of pork shoulder, brisket, or chicken thighs with a bottle of salsa verde. Set it on low and by the time you're back from work, you'll have taco filler waiting for you. Just add corn tortillas and a scoop of guac and you're ready for dinner.

BAKE BETTER BEANS

Slow cookers do more than just main dishes. Cover dried beans with plenty of water, some bay leaves, and a few cloves of garlic and cook for 4 hours on low. The results will make you wonder why you even mess with the canned stuff.

OUR PICK

WEST BEND VERSATILITY COOKER
$79.99 WestBend.com

Browning meat before a braise is a vital step in maximizing flavor of the final dish. The best slow cookers feature pots that transition easily to your stovetop so you can quickly sear meat over high heat before sticking it on for the slow burn. This one does just that. Better still, the programmable timer switches directly into warming mode when the cooking's finished.

POWER TIME HI LO WM GRIDD

The Slow Cooker Matrix

Why cook slowly? Inexpensive cuts of meat also happen to possess an inordinate amount of flavor, but to enjoy it, you first need to break down all the connective tissue in the meat. Steady low temperatures do it best, which is why slow cookers are so useful: Dump a bunch of inexpensive meat and vegetables into the vessel, cover with your choice of liquid, press on, and disappear for 8 hours. One taste and you'll see why slow cookers make culinary geniuses out of people who can't fry an egg.

Four Master Braises

These slow-cooked comfort concoctions span the globe, but all have one thing in common: huge flavor. Crock, lock, and load.

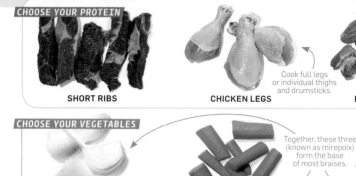

CHOOSE YOUR PROTEIN

SHORT RIBS

CHICKEN LEGS

Cook full legs or individual thighs and drumsticks.

PORK SHOULDER

CHOOSE YOUR VEGETABLES

ONIONS

CARROTS

Together, these three (known as mirepoix) form the base of most braises.

CELERY

CHOOSE YOUR BRAISING LIQUID

RED WINE

WHITE WINE

The flavor of the beer will really affect the final dish, so choose wisely.

BEER

CHOOSE YOUR FLAVOR ENHANCERS

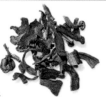

TOMATO PASTE

A few spoonfuls of tomato paste add body and flavor to the braise.

DRIED MUSHROOMS

BAY LEAVES

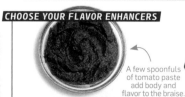

ASIAN SHORT RIBS
Short ribs + onions + carrots + garlic + soy sauce + rice wine vinegar + beef stock + ginger + honey

LAMB OSSOBUCO
Lamb shanks + mirepoix + garlic + red wine + stock + tomato paste + bay leaves

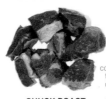

LAMB SHANKS

CHUCK ROAST

Dried beans cook effortlessly this way. Just cook over low for no more than 3 hours.

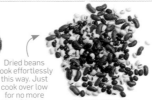

DRIED BEANS

GARLIC

POTATOES

Add vegetables that cook quickly during the last hour of the slow cooker—unless you don't mind eating mush.

MUSHROOMS

Balsamic, wine, rice wine, or sherry

VINEGAR

SOY SAUCE

BEEF OR CHICKEN STOCK

Thyme, rosemary, parsley

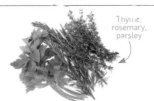

FRESH HERBS

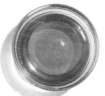

HONEY

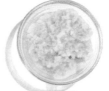

GINGER

COQ AU VIN (RED WINE CHICKEN)
Chicken legs + mirepoix + garlic + red wine + chicken stock + tomato paste + mushrooms

PORK RAGU
Pork shoulder + mirepoix + white wine + stock + can of tomatoes + rosemary

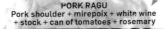

Once cooked, shred the meat with a fork, combine with some of the vegetables and braising liquid, and serve over pasta or polenta.

The Rules of the Braise

Brown the base
Always sear your meat in oil first. The deeper the caramelization, the more flavor the dish will have.

Leave no flavor behind
After you've browned the meat and transferred to the slow cooker, deglaze the cooking pan by adding wine or other liquid and scrape up any bits stuck to the bottom. This will allow you to extract every last bit of flavor left behind by the meat.

Liquify
Use enough liquid (including the liquid from the pan) to cover the meat. Your best bet is to pair at least half stock with another flavorful liquid—wine, beer, vinegar, soy.

Build flavor
Vegetables, spices, and herbs add nuance to the braise. Top and cook on low for 8 hours or on high for 4. All of these recipes (and the other slow cooker recipes in the book) can be done without a slow cooker. Simply place in a 300°F oven until the meat begins to fall apart.

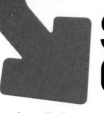

Sunday Roast Chicken

This dish is every bit as delicious on a Tuesday or Friday, but there's something about a chicken roasting on a bed of vegetables that makes the Sunday night specter of the long week ahead that much more palatable. The key to this chicken is seasoning it long before cooking. The salt will penetrate the flesh, seasoning the bird down to the bone and helping create a juicier roast. If you follow no other part of this recipe, at least follow that one trick.

You'll Need:

- 1 whole chicken (about 4 lbs)
- 2 Tbsp fresh thyme leaves
- 1 Tbsp Dijon mustard
- 4 cloves garlic, minced

Grated zest of 1 lemon

- 2 Tbsp olive oil

Salt and black pepper to taste

- 2 medium onions, quartered
- 2 cups peeled and chopped butternut squash
- 4 cups Brussels sprouts, ends removed

The chicken can be roasted with any firm vegetables: potatoes, carrots, parsnips, turnips. Vary at will; just be sure to cut into equal pieces.

How to Make It:

- The morning of the day you roast the chicken, rinse it and pat it dry. Combine the thyme, mustard, garlic, lemon zest, and 1 tablespoon olive oil and rub over the chicken. Season the chicken with salt and black pepper. Refrigerate until you're ready to cook, up to 12 hours.

- Preheat the oven to 425°F. Place the vegetables in a large roasting pan. Add the remaining 1 tablespoon olive oil, plus salt and pepper, and toss. Use kitchen twine to tie the chicken legs together with a knot at the end of the drumsticks. Use another piece of twine to tie the wings together tight against the body of the chicken by looping the string around the wing tip, then running it under the chicken back.

- Place the chicken in the roasting pan and roast on the middle rack for 45 to 55 minutes, until the skin is deeply browned and an instant-read thermometer inserted into the thigh registers 170°F.

- Rest the chicken for 10 minutes before carving and serving with the vegetables.

Makes 4 servings

Per Serving

$3.07

520 calories
27 g fat
(7 g saturated)
820 mg sodium

Master THE **TECHNIQUE**

Pan Gravy

A roast chicken leaves behind the perfect base for a rich gravy. Combine the roasting juices accumulated beneath the chicken in a pan with a spoonful of flour. Slowly add warm chicken stock, whisking to keep lumps from forming. Flavor with herbs, a splash of white wine, or a squeeze of lemon.

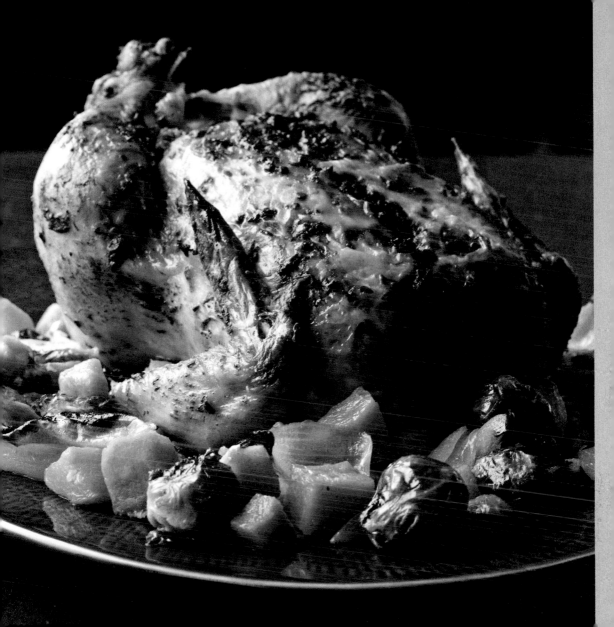

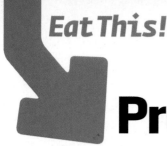

Provençal Chicken

This is the type of simple, healthy, satisfying dish that gives Mediterranean cooking its reputation as the perfect fusion of flavor and nutrition. All of the key components—white wine, tomatoes, olives, herbs—have the distinct advantage of being both intensely flavorful and incredibly good for you. Truth be told, we're not really sure if people in Provence eat their chicken like this, but it has the soul of southern France in every bite.

You'll Need:

- 1 Tbsp olive oil
- 8 boneless, skinless chicken thighs (about 1½ lb total)
- Salt and black pepper to taste
- 1 small yellow onion, minced
- 3 cloves garlic, minced
- 3 Roma tomatoes, diced
- 1 cup dry white wine
- 1 cup chicken stock
- 1 tsp herbes de Provence
- ¼ cup pitted Kalamata olives, roughly chopped
- Fresh basil for garnish (optional)

How to Make It:

- Heat the olive oil in a large sauté pan over medium-high heat. Season the chicken all over with salt and black pepper. Add the chicken to the pan and cook, turning once, for about 6 minutes total, until seared and nicely browned. (Work in two batches if need be, so as not to overcrowd the pan.) Remove the chicken to a plate and reserve.

- To the same pan, add the onions, garlic, and tomatoes and cook for about 5 minutes, until the onions and tomatoes are very soft. Add the wine, broth, and herbes de Provence and bring the mixture to a simmer. Return the chicken to the pan and simmer uncovered, turning the chicken halfway through, for about 20 minutes, until the meat is very tender. Stir in the olives, garnish with basil if you like, and serve.

Makes 4 servings

Per Serving
$2.77
340 calories
15 g fat
(2.5 g saturated)
680 mg sodium

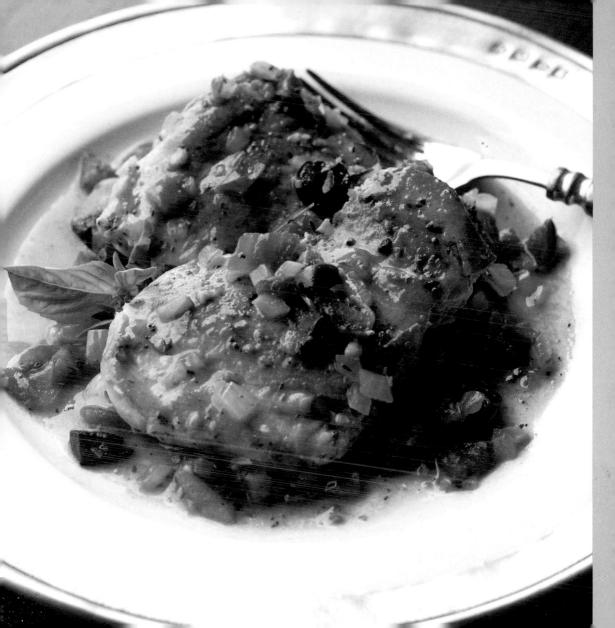

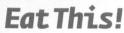

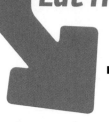

Turkey Meat Loaf

Among the most comforting of all comfort foods, a well-made meat loaf delivers that warm, rib-sticking goodness we all crave. The key to excellent meat loaf is threefold: a well-seasoned base, a generous glaze, and careful cooking. We realize that some people may still bear scars from the bone-dry loaves of their childhoods, but this creation will banish those with a single bite.

You'll Need:

TURKEY MEAT LOAF

1 small onion, peeled and quartered

½ red bell pepper, stemmed and quartered

1 small carrot, peeled and roughly chopped

2 cloves garlic, peeled

1½ lb ground turkey

½ cup bread crumbs

¼ cup low-sodium chicken stock

1 egg, beaten

1 Tbsp Worcestershire

1 Tbsp low-sodium soy sauce

½ tsp dried thyme

½ tsp salt

½ tsp black pepper

GLAZE

½ cup ketchup

2 Tbsp brown sugar

2 Tbsp low-sodium soy sauce

2 Tbsp apple cider vinegar

How to Make It:

● Preheat the oven to 325°F.

● Combine the onion, bell pepper, carrot, and garlic in a food processor and pulse until finely minced. (If you don't have a food processor, you can do this by hand.) Combine the vegetables with the turkey, bread crumbs, stock, egg, Worcestershire, soy sauce, thyme, and salt and black pepper in a large mixing bowl. Gently mix until all of the ingredients are evenly distributed.

● Dump the meat loaf mixture into a 13" x 9" baking dish and use your hands to form a loaf roughly 9" long and 6" wide. Mix the glaze ingredients together and spread over the meat loaf. Bake for 1 hour, until the glaze has turned a deep shade of red and an instant-read thermometer inserted into the center of the loaf registers 160°F.

Makes 6 servings

LEFTOVER♥LOVE

There are more than a few ways to reinvent meat loaf the next day (topped with a fried egg, covered with sautéed peppers and onions), but for our money, the best bet is still a thick meat loaf sandwich. Gently sauté onions until nicely caramelized while reheating the meat loaf in a 325°F oven with a thin slice of smoked gouda, and serve it all on a toasted bun. It's worth making this recipe for the sandwich alone.

Per Serving
$1.73
290 calories
11 g fat
(3 g saturated)
920 mg sodium

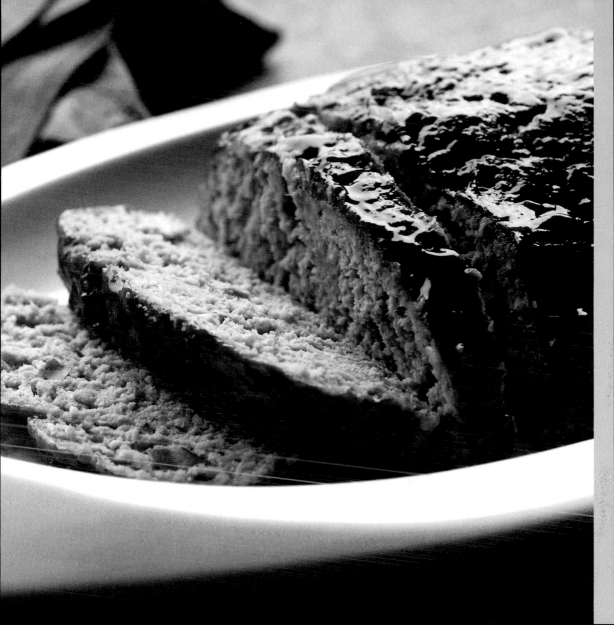

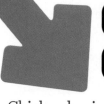

Eat This!

Creamy Mushroom Chicken

Chicken buried in mushrooms and cream is the type of dish as at home in a country kitchen as it is in an upscale urban restaurant. We take cues from both ends of the spectrum: brown mushrooms and chicken stock from the country, a touch of sherry and some dried mushrooms from the city. The combination of Greek yogurt and half-and-half gives the sauce richness and a lovely velvety texture without weighing it down.

You'll Need:

- 1 Tbsp olive oil, plus more if needed
- 4 small boneless skinless chicken breasts (6 oz each)

Salt and black pepper to taste

- 1 medium shallot, minced
- 3 cloves garlic, minced
- 8 oz cremini mushrooms, sliced
- ¼ cup sherry •
- ¼ cup dried mushrooms (porcini, chanterelle, shiitake), soaked in ½ cup warm water for 15 minutes
- ½ cup low-sodium chicken stock
- ¼ cup half-and-half
- ¼ cup Greek yogurt

How to Make It:

- Heat the olive oil over high heat in a large sauté pan. Season the chicken all over with salt and black pepper. Add the chicken to the pan and sear for about 3 minutes, until a nice deep brown crust develops on the bottom sides. Flip and continue to cook for 3 minutes longer, until the other sides are also nicely browned. Remove to a plate.

- If the pan is dry after cooking the chicken, add a thin film of olive oil. Add the shallot, garlic, and cremini mushrooms to the pan and sauté for about 3 minutes, until the mushrooms are lightly browned. Season with salt and black pepper. Add the sherry and cook for 1 minute, using a spatula or wooden spoon to scrape loose any browned bits from the bottom of the pan. Add the dried mushrooms (and soaking liquid), chicken stock, and half-and-half. Turn the heat down to low and return the chicken to the pan.

- Continue cooking for 8 to 10 minutes, until the liquid reduces by half and the chicken is cooked through. Add the yogurt and stir to create a smooth, uniform sauce. Divide the chicken among 4 plates and top with the mushroom sauce.

Makes 4 servings

In a pinch, sweet, fortified wines like Madeira or Marsala will work in place of the sherry.

Per Serving
$3.46
270 calories
10 g fat
(3 g saturated)
420 mg sodium

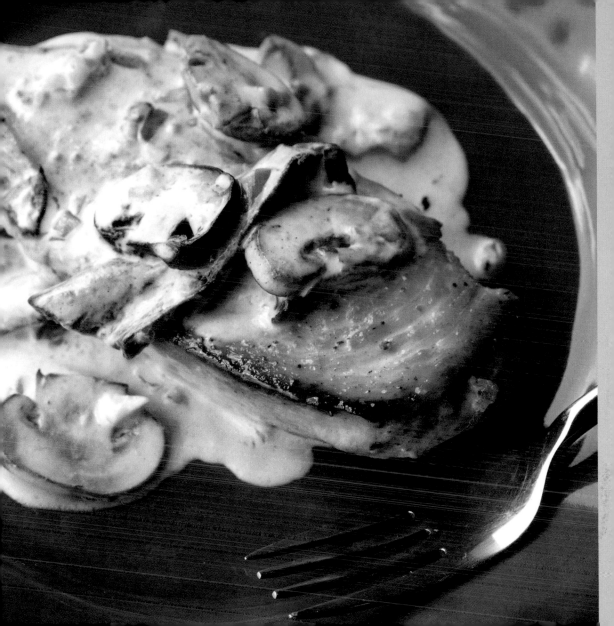

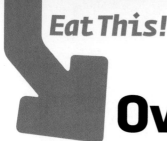

Oven-Fried Chicken

We'll be the first to admit that the idea of oven-fried chicken rubs us the wrong way. Usually the chicken comes out dry and the crust soggy or non-existent, leaving your need to eat crispy, juicy food unfulfilled. But this version defies all expectations. First, the chicken is brined in buttermilk and hot sauce, then it's coated in bread crumbs that have been tossed in a gentle amount of oil. The result? The juiciest, crispiest oven-fried chicken ever.

You'll Need:

- 8 chicken drumsticks
- 4 cups nonfat buttermilk
- ¼ cup salt
- ¼ cup sugar
- 1 Tbsp hot sauce (preferably Frank's RedHot pepper sauce)
- 2 cups panko bread crumbs
- 2 Tbsp canola or vegetable oil
- 1 tsp chili powder
- ½ tsp garlic salt

How to Make It:

- Combine the chicken, buttermilk, salt, sugar, and hot sauce in a sealable plastic bag and shake to combine. Refrigerate for at least 2 hours or up to 12 hours.

- Preheat the oven to 350°F.

- In a large mixing bowl, use your fingers to break up the panko bread crumbs into slightly smaller pieces (this will help create a more even coating on the chicken). Add the oil, chili powder, and garlic salt and stir to combine. Working with one piece at a time, remove the chicken from the marinade, shake off the excess liquid, then toss in the bread crumbs until thoroughly coated.

- Place the chicken pieces on a rack set in a rimmed nonstick baking sheet. Bake on the middle rack of the oven for about 30 minutes, until the bread crumbs are evenly browned and the chicken is cooked through.

Makes 4 servings

Per Serving
$1.89
250 calories
14 g fat
(3 g saturated)
620 mg sodium

LEFTOVER♥LOVE

Nothing quite like coming to the fridge at midnight with a case of the munchies and finding a pile of cold fried chicken to dive into. With this low-cal chicken, for once it's a safe move, but still, we implore you to keep the chicken around long enough to try one of these other dishes.

- Flaky Southern Biscuits (page 60) with chicken (pulled off the bone for this and the following recipes), honey, and hot sauce
- Mixed green salad with chicken, toasted walnuts, diced apple, blue cheese, and balsamic vinaigrette
- BLT with chunks of chicken

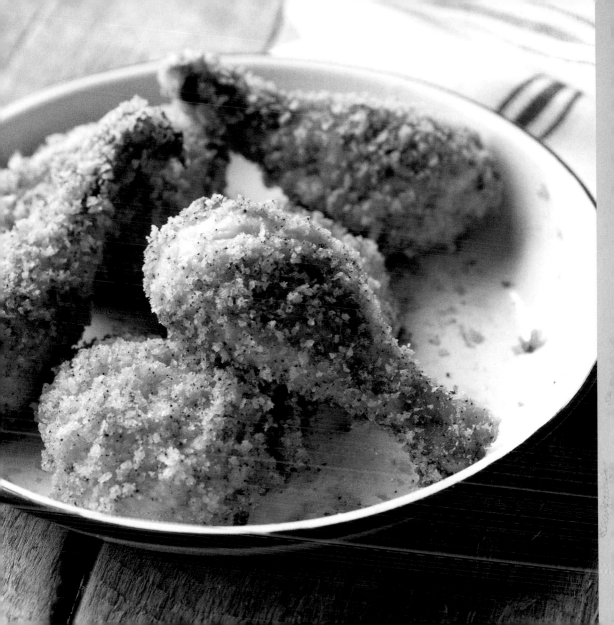

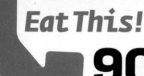

Eat This!

90-Minute Roasted Turkey

with Orange-Cranberry Relish

This magical turkey came about out of sheer necessity. It was Matt's senior year in college and a spontaneous Thanksgiving feast had materialized around him. The only problem? It was 7 p.m. and there was no turkey in the oven. He remembered an old recipe espousing the joys of a turkey blasted at 500°F, effectively searing the skin a beautiful brown and leaving the meat moist inside. By 9 p.m., one of the greatest Thanksgiving spreads on record was laid before a group of 20 hungry students. This bird was the centerpiece.

You'll Need:

1 (12–14 lb) turkey

1 Tbsp kosher salt

Orange-Cranberry Relish (page 318)

It's important that the turkey be this size. Larger turkeys will burn on the surface before being cooked all the way through.

Per Serving

$1.29

260 calories

6 g fat
(2.5 g saturated)

240 mg sodium

How to Make It:

- The morning before you plan to cook the turkey, season the bird all over with the salt.

- Ninety minutes before cooking the turkey, remove it from the fridge so it can come up to room temperature. Thirty minutes before cooking, drape a sealable plastic bag filled with ice over the breasts. (Sounds crazy, but the ice will cool the breasts and help prevent them from overcooking while the dark meat cooks through.)

- Preheat the oven to 500°F. Place the turkey on a roasting rack set in a large roasting pan. Roast the turkey on the bottom rack of the oven until the skin is deeply bronzed and an instant-read thermometer inserted into the deepest part of a thigh registers 160°F. (If the wing tips or ends of the drumsticks begin to burn, you can cover them with foil.) This will take anywhere between 75 and 100 minutes, depending on the size of your turkey and the heat of your oven.

Makes about 15 servings

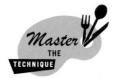

Master THE **TECHNIQUE**

Because of the high heat used to cook this turkey, you may get a bit of smoke in your oven. The best way to curtail the smoke, of course, is to have a clean oven. Beyond that, cover the wing tips and the drumstick ends midway through the cooking, as they may char when exposed to high heat for so long. If this sounds like a pain in the butt, remember that you'll be cooking one of the best turkeys of your life in just 90 minutes.

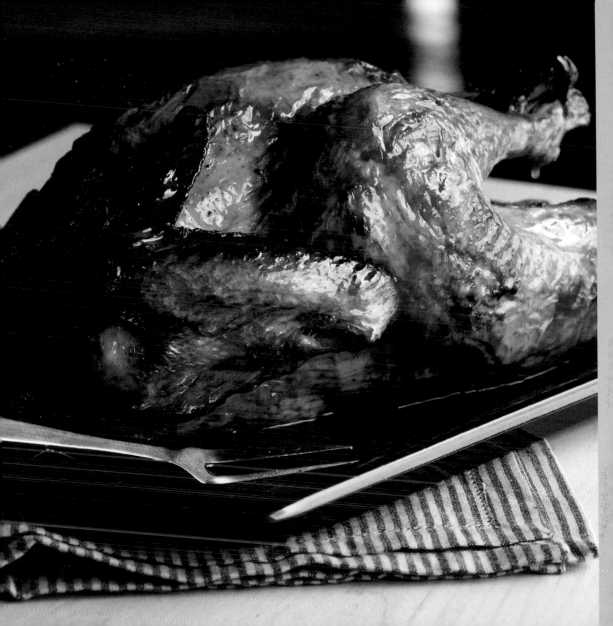

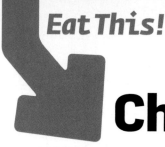
Chicken Parm

Despite the fact that it's the size of a Frisbee, fried in oil, and covered in cheese, the biggest problem with chicken parm remains the pile of pasta upon which it invariably is served. That's why we serve our chicken parm with garlicky spinach: It not only cuts calories and boosts nutrition dramatically, it also adds a citrus punch that pairs perfectly with the saucy chicken. We coat the bird in Japanese-style bread crumbs (which crisp up better than the standard variety) and then bake it until golden brown, a move that saves you the hassle (and the unwanted fat) of frying at home.

You'll Need:

- 1 extra-large egg
- 2 cups panko bread crumbs
- ¼ cup grated Parmesan cheese
- 1 tsp olive oil
- 1 tsp Italian seasoning
- Salt and black pepper to taste
- 4 small boneless, skinless chicken breasts (6 oz each), pounded to uniform ⅓-inch thickness
- 1½ cups Tomato Sauce (page 321), heated
- ½ cup shredded mozzarella cheese
- Garlic-Lemon Spinach (page 312)

How to Make It:

- Preheat the oven to 400°F.
- Crack the egg into a shallow dish and beat. In a separate shallow dish (a pie pan works nicely), combine the bread crumbs, Parmesan, olive oil, Italian seasoning, and a few generous pinches of salt and black pepper.
- Working with one piece of chicken at a time, dip into the egg, then into the bread crumbs, using your fingers to press the crumbs into the chicken. Place the chicken breasts on a baking sheet or roasting pan and place in the oven on the middle rack. Bake for about 12 minutes, until the chicken is firm to the touch and the bread crumbs are golden brown.
- Remove the chicken from the oven and set the oven to broil. Cover each breast with a good ladle of tomato sauce and a handful of mozzarella. Return to the middle rack of the oven and broil for about 3 minutes, until the cheese is melted and bubbling.
- Serve the chicken over the spinach with extra tomato sauce, if you like.

Makes 4 servings

Per Serving
$3.13
340 calories
9 g fat
(3.5 g saturated)
540 mg sodium

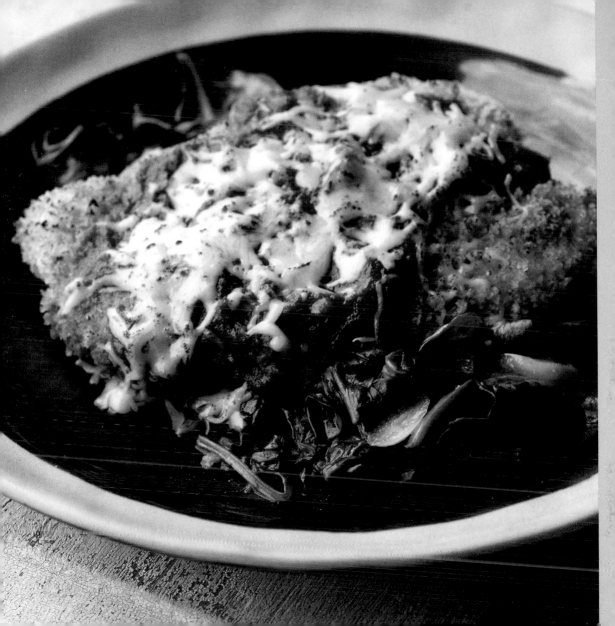

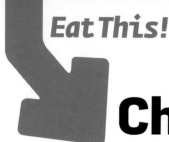

Eat This!

Chicken Potpie

Potpies may be one of America's favorite comfort foods, but there's nothing comforting about a dish that can swallow up an entire day's worth of calories, fat, and sodium, as some restaurant renditions do. We teach you a few simple tricks for creating a deeply delicious, remarkably lean potpie.

You'll Need:

- 2 Tbsp butter
- 1 onion, chopped
- 2 carrots, chopped
- 2 cloves garlic, minced
- 2 cups stemmed and quartered white or cremini mushrooms
- 2 cups frozen pearl onions
- 2 cups chopped cooked chicken (leftover or pulled from a store-bought rotisserie chicken)
- ¼ cup flour
- 2 cups low-sodium chicken broth, warmed
- 1 cup 2% or whole milk
- ½ cup half-and-half
- 1½ cups frozen peas
- Salt and black pepper to taste
- 1 sheet puff pastry, defrosted
- 2 egg whites, lightly beaten

How to Make It:

- Heat the butter in a large saucepan over medium heat. Cook the onion, carrots, and garlic until softened, about 5 minutes. Add the mushrooms and pearl onions and cook, stirring occasionally, for another 5 minutes. Stir in the chicken and the flour.

- Slowly add in the chicken broth, whisking to avoid clumping (having the broth warm helps smooth out the sauce). Add the milk and half-and-half and simmer for 10 to 15 minutes, until the sauce has thickened and lightly clings to the vegetables and chicken. Stir in the peas. Season with salt and pepper.

- Preheat the oven to 375°F. Cut the pastry into quarters. Roll out each piece on a floured surface to make a 6" square. Divide the chicken mixture among 4 ovenproof bowls. (Or pour chicken in a 13 x 9-inch baking dish and top with a single ¼-inch-thick piece of pastry.) Place a pastry square over the top of each bowl and trim away the excess with a paring knife; pinch the dough around the edges of the bowl to secure it. Brush the tops with the egg whites and bake until golden brown, about 25 minutes.

Makes 4 servings

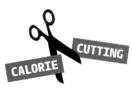

CALORIE CUTTING

The bulk of the calories in potpies come from the butter-laden pastry that crowns the bowls. This recipe calls for puff pastry rolled extra thin to minimize the caloric impact—but to further reduce your fat intake, you can make two quick substitutions: 1) Instead of puff pastry, try a few layers of phyllo dough brushed with a bit of butter. 2) Replace the half-and-half with another ½ cup milk.

Per Serving
$3.84
350 calories
15 g fat
(8 g saturated)
650 mg sodium

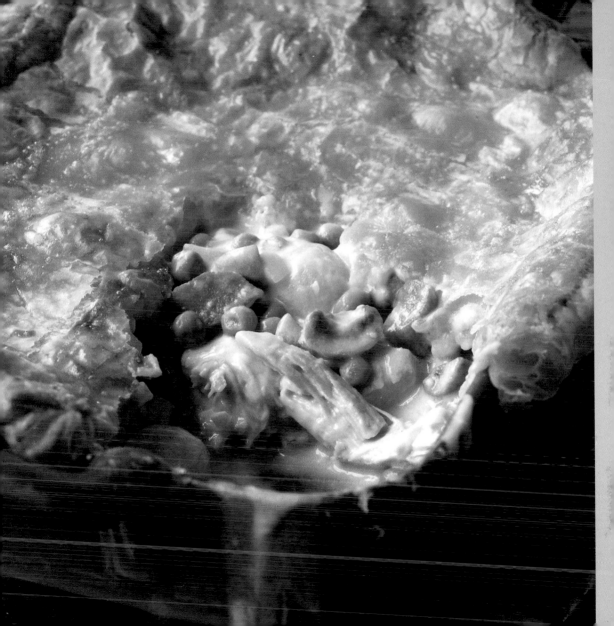

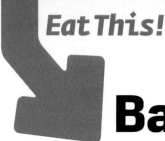

Eat This!

Basque Chicken

The Basques of northern Spain have long taken pride in their prodigious culinary powers. After all, this is the land of powerful wines, pintxos (an early form of tapas), and San Sebastián, one of the great gastronomic cities of the world. This dish combines some of the great flavors of northern Spain—smoked paprika, sweet peppers, piquant chorizo—in a slow-cooked stew that could warm even the most frigid soul. We've taken a few liberties with the flavors here (dark beer isn't exactly a Spanish staple), but the results reflect the beauty of the Basque kitchen.

You'll Need:

1 Tbsp olive oil

4 bone-in, skin-on chicken breasts

Salt and black pepper to taste

1 link Spanish chorizo, sliced into ¼"-thick coins

1 bottle (12 oz) porter, stout, or other dark beer

1½ cups low-sodium chicken stock

2 Tbsp sherry vinegar or red wine vinegar

1 large onion, quartered

1 red bell pepper, chopped

8 cloves garlic, peeled

1 tsp smoked paprika

½ tsp cumin

2 bay leaves

4 cups baby spinach (optional)

How to Make It:

● Heat the olive oil in a large cast-iron skillet or sauté pan over medium-high heat. Season the chicken all over with salt and black pepper and cook the pieces until browned on all sides, about 7 minutes. Add the chorizo and continue cooking for another 2 minutes, until the chorizo has browned as well. Transfer the meat to the slow cooker.

● Pour the beer into the skillet, scraping the bottom to loosen any brown bits. Add to the slow cooker, along with the stock, vinegar, onion, bell pepper, garlic, paprika, cumin, and bay leaves and cook on low for 4 hours.

● If using spinach, add it 10 minutes before serving, giving it enough time to cook down in the warm braising liquid. Before serving, discard the bay leaves and taste and adjust the seasoning with salt and black pepper. Serve in wide shallow bowls with a ladle of the braising liquid poured over the top.

Makes 4 servings

Per Serving
$3.42
370 calories
20 g fat
(6 g saturated)
700 mg sodium

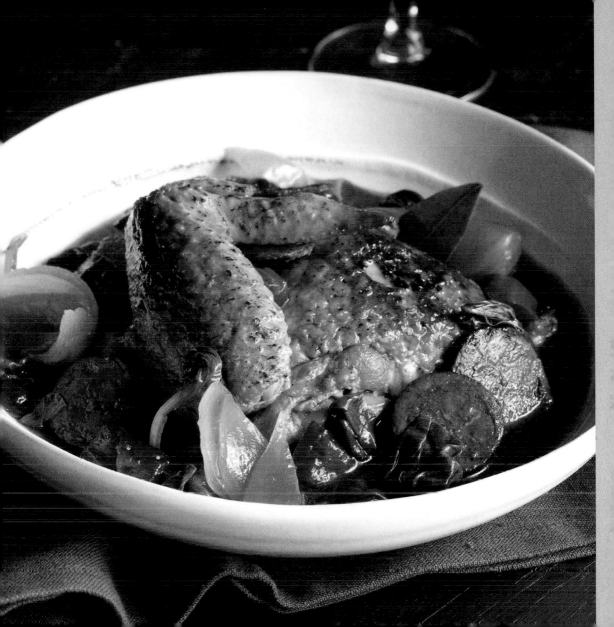

Jambalaya

No city or region in America lays claim to a richer, more influential lineup of culinary creations than New Orleans and the surrounding Creole country. Gumbo, étouffée, beignets, po'boys—all are part of Louisiana's incomparable culinary heritage. No dish, though, is more famous than jambalaya, the rice-based hodgepodge of meat, seafood, and vegetables not unlike the Spanish paella. By decreasing the rice ratio and increasing the produce and protein, this recipe cuts the calories and carbs dramatically. But it still has enough soul to satisfy the most discerning Creole critics.

You'll Need:

- 1 tsp olive or canola oil
- 1 cup diced turkey kielbasa
- 1 medium onion, diced
- 1 medium green bell pepper, diced
- 2 cloves garlic, minced
- 8 oz boneless, skinless chicken breast, cut into ½" cubes
- 1 cup long-grain rice
- 2¼ cups low-sodium chicken stock
- 1 can (14 oz) diced tomatoes
- 1 Tbsp tomato paste
- ⅛ tsp cayenne
- 2 bay leaves
- 8 oz medium shrimp, peeled and deveined
- Salt and black pepper to taste
- Frank's RedHot, Tabasco, or other hot sauce
- Chopped scallions (optional)

How to Make It:

- Heat the oil in a large skillet or saute pan over medium heat. Add the kielbasa and cook for about 3 minutes, until lightly browned. Add the onion, bell pepper, and garlic and cook, stirring occasionally, for 4 to 5 minutes, until the vegetables have softened.
- Push the vegetables and kielbasa to the perimeter, making a well in the center of the pan. Add the chicken and sauté until lightly browned but not cooked through, about 3 minutes. Stir in the rice, stock, tomatoes, tomato paste, cayenne, and bay leaves. Turn the heat to low, cover, and simmer for 17 minutes, until nearly all of the liquid has been absorbed by the rice. Uncover, add the shrimp, and cook for 2 to 3 minutes, until the rice is tender and the shrimp is cooked through. Discard the bay leaves. Season with salt, black pepper, and hot sauce and garnish with the scallions, if using.

Makes 4 servings

Per Serving
$4.15
380 calories
15 g fat
(4.5 g saturated)
1,070 mg sodium

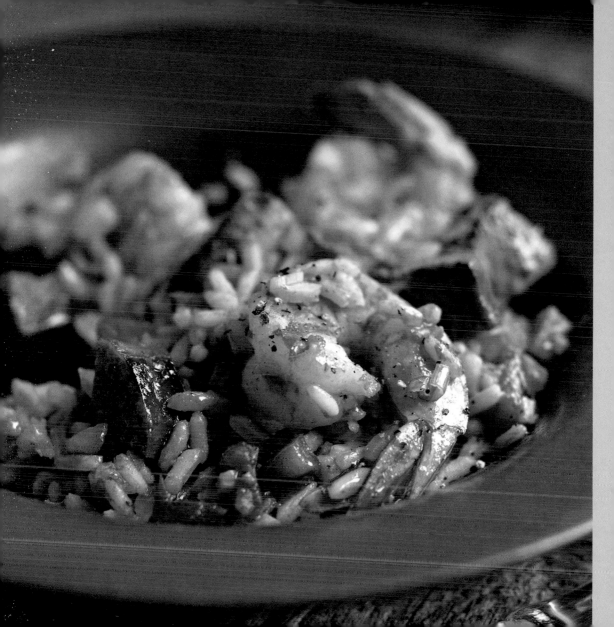

Chicken & Dumplings

This is the kind of food Mom makes when the sniffles set in. It has many of the same magical powers and core flavors of chicken noodle soup—root vegetables, savory broth, shredded chicken—but is made more substantial by the addition of a roux to thicken the soup base and, of course, fluffy dumplings. Of course, the real magic is in those pillows of rosemary-scented joy, which soak up the hearty liquid and, when combined with the juicy chicken, make for one of the most satisfying, savory bites imaginable.

You'll Need:

- 2 Tbsp butter
- 4 medium carrots, diced
- 1 medium onion, diced
- 3 Tbsp plus ⅔ cup flour
- ½ tsp dried thyme
- 4 cups low-sodium chicken stock
- 1 lb boneless, skinless chicken thighs
- Salt and black pepper to taste
- 1½ tsp baking powder
- 1 tsp chopped fresh rosemary
- ½ cup 2% milk
- ½ cup frozen peas

How to Make It:

- Heat the butter in a pot or large saucepan over medium heat. Add the carrots and onions and cook for about 5 minutes, until softened. Add the 3 tablespoons flour and the thyme, stirring so that the vegetables are evenly coated. Slowly add the stock, whisking to prevent lumps from forming. Bring to a gentle simmer.

- Season the chicken thighs with salt and black pepper and add to the pot, submerging them in the stock. Poach the chicken for about 8 minutes, until just cooked through. Remove to a cutting board to rest.

- Combine the remaining ⅔ cup flour with the baking powder, rosemary, ¼ teaspoon salt, and lots of black pepper. Add the milk and gently stir until the dough just comes together. Form loosely into 8 dumplings and drop them directly into the soup. Cover the pot and cook over low heat for 10 minutes, until the dumplings have firmed up.

- Shred the reserved chicken. Add to the pot, along with the peas, stirring carefully so as not to break up the dumplings. Heat through for 1 minute before serving.

Makes 4 servings

Per Serving
$1.83
380 calories
12 g fat
(5 g saturated)
810 mg sodium

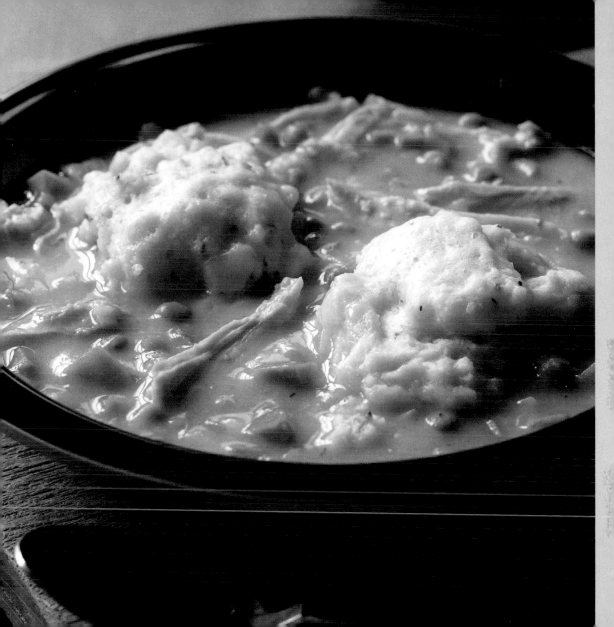

CHAPTER 8

REDMEAT

America's Worst RED MEAT

WORST CHILI
Steak 'n Shake's Chili Deluxe (bowl)

1,220 calories
74 g fat
(39 g saturated, 1.5 g trans)
2,560 mg sodium
Price: $3.99

"Chili" is short for chili con carne—a Mexican stew anchored by chile peppers, beef, and onions. "Chili Deluxe" is short for beef con ab flab. Fattier cuts of meat may come at a higher cost to your health, but they also come with a lower price tag, which is why most restaurant chili is brimming with subpar beef. And Steak 'n Shake takes the fat frenzy one step further by topping its chili with a fistful of shredded cheese. Our suggestion for ensuring your bowl doesn't house half a day's calories: Keep your meat where you can see it—in your home fridge.

Eat This Instead!
Crockpot Chili (page 212)

250 calories
8 g fat (2.5 g saturated)
500 mg sodium
Cost per serving: $1.80
Save! 970 calories and $2.19!

WORST PORK CHOPS
Cheesecake Factory's Grilled Pork Chops

1,370 calories
N/A g fat
(39 g saturated)
2,400 mg sodium
Price: $19.95

Don't blame the pig. An 8-ounce center-cut chop—the same cut proudly touted on the Cheesecake Factory menu—contains just 440 calories. After all, this remarkable leanness is one of the many reasons we love pork so much. But no cut is safe in the hands of the

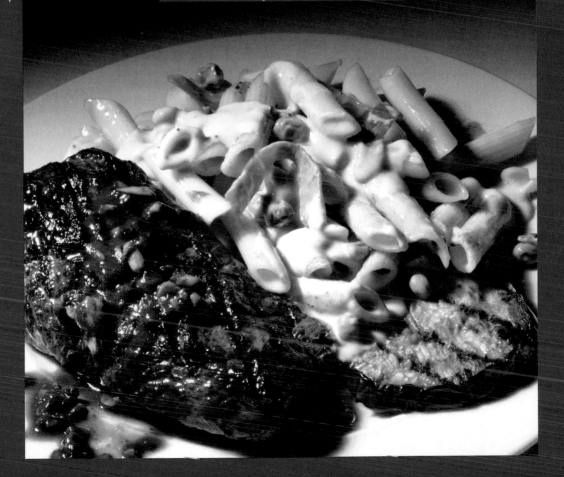

87 grams of fat

A steak is normally a pretty safe menu bet, unless, of course, it's the Chianti BBQ Steak from Macaroni Grill.

restaurant industry, especially those of its most diabolical practitioner, the Cheesecake Factory. The chain keeps its sinful culinary secrets under lock and key, but we're guessing this pork's pitiful performance is owed to a frying pan full of oil and the Factory's typical elephantine portions.

Eat This Instead!
Smothered Pork Chops
(page 210)

260 calories
15 g fat (6 g saturated)
720 mg sodium
Cost per serving: $2.49
Save! 1,110 calories and $17.46!

WORST BURRITO
On The Border's Big Steak Bordurrito (without side salad)

1,550 calories
77 g fat (25 g saturated)
3,210 mg sodium
Price: $10.99

A burrito by any other name would look as bleak. Call it what you will, but the Tex-Mex staple is just an excuse for chains to take as much meat, cheese, rice, and other high-cal fillers as possible, and wrap 'em up in a massive blanket of processed carbs. To take a bad thing and make it worse, On the Border decides to boil the whole burrito in oil. We like our burritos big but not bursting, saucy but not soaking, and lightly toasted, not deep-fried in fat. (That's why we eat them at home, not at a dodgy chain!)

Eat This Instead!
Carne Asada Burritos (page 226)

420 calories
20 g fat (6 g saturated)
660 mg sodium
Cost per serving: $3.37
Save! 1,130 calories and $7.62!

WORST STEAK
Romano's Macaroni Grill's Chianti BBQ Steak

1,460 calories
87 g fat
(43 g saturated, 2g trans)
3,130 mg sodium
Price: $21.00

Despite its association with decadence, steak is often the safest choice at your local restaurant—especially when opting for a lean cut like flank or sirloin. But the problem here isn't the cut (Macaroni Grill uses sirloin cap); it's the size of the steak (roughly as big as a catcher's mitt), the smothering of sugary barbecue sauce, and the shameless sideshow of mac and cheese, bread, and creamy garlic dip. A potent reminder that no steak is as good—or as healthy—as the one you grill yourself.

Eat This Instead!
Steak with Red Wine Sauce (page 222)

380 calories
18 g fat (6 g saturated)
410 mg sodium
Cost per serving: $3.92
Save! 1,080 calories and $17.08!

WORST RIBS
Chili's House BBQ Ribs (full rack without fries)

1,440 calories
107g fat
(41 g saturated)
2,180 mg sodium
Price: $16.99

Ribs are an inherently precarious pork option at any chain. First, they're one of the fattiest cuts the pig has to offer. Second, restaurants make a habit of slathering their racks with sickeningly sweet sauces that contribute tons of superfluous calories. And finally, salt is often the seasoning of choice at big chains, a cheap move that, at Chili's, results in a slab of meat with more than 2 days' worth of sodium! But don't fret: We've developed a two-step process that produces tender, succulent ribs for less than a quarter of the calories.

Eat This Instead!
Smoky Ribs with Peach BBQ Sauce (page 218)

410 calories
31 g fat (11 g saturated)
460 mg sodium
Cost per serving: $2.76
Save! 1,030 calories and $14.23!

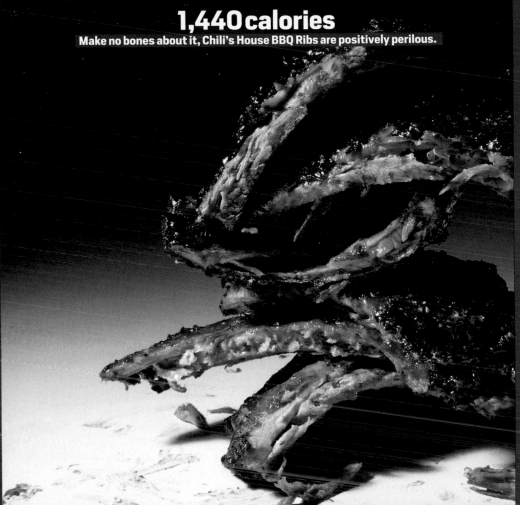

1,440 calories
Make no bones about it, Chili's House BBQ Ribs are positively perilous.

Cast-Iron Skillet

Life would be easier if there were one pan capable of handling all kitchen jobs. There isn't. But if there were, there's no question what metal would form the base of that pan: iron.

For much of history, iron was all anybody needed for cooking. Only in modern times have alternative materials like steel and anodized aluminum come into fashion. Those metals make good (not to mention extremely expensive) pans, but they don't touch the durability and heat distribution of iron. A well-cared-for cast-iron skillet can sear steaks for decades without showing any signs of fatigue.

And while Teflon relies on polytetrafluoroethylene to prevent sticking, cast iron does the same thing naturally, converting the oils from foods cooked in the skillet into a smooth nonstick patina. The metal retains seasoning between uses, meaning you can brown burgers and sauté vegetables with little or no oil at all and still get the caramelization we all crave.

Maintaining a well-seasoned skillet is what scares some people away from cast iron. Listen to the cast-iron evangelicals (yes, they exist), and you might think that cast iron will explode if it touches soap or water. Not so. It's perfectly acceptable to rinse it after each use, and a touch of soap is fine for removing sticky gunk. Just wipe it dry, stick it back in the cupboard, and you'll never have to replace it.

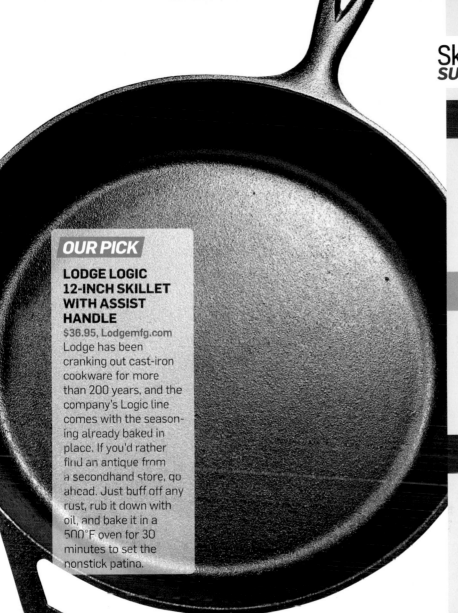

Skillet SUPERPOWERS

SEAR A STEAK INTO SUBMISSION

No cookware retains heat as well as cast iron, which makes it ideal for searing steaks and burgers, browning chicken breasts, and blackening catfish. The thinner the cut, the higher the heat needed to obtain a crust without drying out the meat: For fish, you want the heat on at full blast; for a thick steak, you'll want to maintain a medium flame.

WOK THIS WAY

Its heat-holding ability makes a cast-iron skillet the perfect stand-in for a wok. Heat a thin film of oil over high heat and cook minced garlic, ginger, and scallions for 30 seconds. Stir in your chopped vegetables and protein, stir-fry until the meat is cooked through, then splash in soy sauce and sriracha.

BUILD A BETTER BREAKFAST

Bacon and sausage are the obvious breakfast candidates, but cast iron creates beautiful brown crusts on pancakes and French toast. And because a well-kept skillet develops a natural nonstick sheen, you can fry an egg with just a few drops of oil.

OUR PICK

LODGE LOGIC 12-INCH SKILLET WITH ASSIST HANDLE

$36.95, Lodgemfg.com
Lodge has been cranking out cast-iron cookware for more than 200 years, and the company's Logic line comes with the seasoning already baked in place. If you'd rather find an antique from a secondhand store, go ahead. Just buff off any rust, rub it down with oil, and bake it in a 500°F oven for 30 minutes to set the nonstick patina.

The Meatball Matrix

Meatballs are hardly the sole province of Italian grandmothers and their burbling vats of tomato gravy. In fact, few foods transcend geographic barriers as deliciously as the meatball does, and many of the world's food cultures have molded it to their culinary wills. Here is a road map to meatball creation, along with a few tricks to help you nail the craft. Don't worry—when it comes to meatballs, even the experiments turn out pretty darn delicious.

Four Master Meatballs

The true genius of the meatball is its infinite versatility. This chart only scratches the surface of the flavor potential. Follow the basic formula, but dig through the pantry to stretch the boundaries.

CHOOSE A GROUND PROTEIN *(1½ pounds total)*

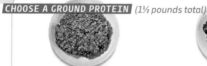

PORK   **BEEF**   **TURKEY**

STANDARD BINDER

For extra-moist meatballs, tear a baguette or sliced bread into large crumbs and soak in milk for 10 minutes. Squeeze the milk out before adding to the mix.

2 LARGE EGGS   **¾ CUP PLAIN DRY BREAD CRUMBS**

CHOOSE FILLERS

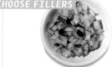

For more bite, add raw onions and garlic, but make sure they're finely minced (or grated on a cheese grater). For a gentler effect, sauté in olive oil until soft before adding.

MINCED ONION   **MINCED GARLIC**

CHOOSE HERBS AND SPICES

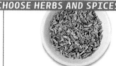

FENNEL SEEDS   **RED PEPPER FLAKES**   **GRATED CITRUS ZEST**

CHOOSE A SAUCE

In a medium saucepan, combine 2 tablespoons olive oil, ½ minced onion, 2 cloves minced garlic, and ¼ teaspoon red pepper flakes. Sauté until the onion is soft, then add one 28-ounce can whole tomatoes, breaking up the tomatoes with a fork. Simmer for about 15 minutes, until the sauce thickens.

Simmer 2 cups chopped mango with ½ cup orange juice, ¼ cup minced red onion, 1 tablespoon minced jalapeño, and 2 cloves minced garlic for 20 minutes.

TOMATO SAUCE   **MANGO CHUTNEY**

SPICY LAMB MEATBALLS
Binder + lamb + red pepper flakes + fresh mint or parsley, with Tomato Sauce

TUNA SATAY MEATBALLS
Binder + tuna + ginger + garlic + cilantro, with Thai Peanut Sauce

LAMB

Remove the skin and bones, and pulse in a food processor until the flesh is reduced to small, pebble-sized pieces.

TUNA OR SALMON

Meatball Magic

To make your masterpiece, combine the Standard Binder with any combination of protein and sidekicks, form into golf ball–size meatballs, and bake in a 400°F for about 20 minutes, until nicely browned on the outside and just cooked through. Simmer in the sauce for 15 minutes before serving, or serve as is with the sauce on the side.

GRATED GINGER

GRATED PARMESAN

MINCED JALAPEÑO

CUMIN

FRESH HERBS (PARSLEY, CILANTRO, BASIL, MINT)

Sauté ½ pound sliced white or cremini mushrooms until browned. Stir in 2 tablespoons flour. Slowly pour in 2 cups broth, whisking to prevent lumps. Stir in ¼ cup heavy cream and simmer until the gravy has thickened.

MUSHROOM GRAVY

Combine 2 tablespoons each Thai red curry paste and peanut butter with 1 cup of coconut milk and the juice of a lime. Simmer for 5 minutes.

THAI PEANUT SAUCE

MANGO PORK MEATBALLS
Binder + pork + ginger + garlic + jalapeño, with Mango Chutney

MEATBALLS IN MUSHROOM GRAVY
Binder + beef + onion + garlic + allspice, with Mushroom Gravy

The Rules of the Meatball

1. Make it moist
Eggs, ricotta, and milk-soaked bread crumbs all add moisture. Forming the balls should be messy; if the mixture isn't sticky, then your meatballs will be dry.

2. Season to perfection
Proper seasoning—especially with salt—is paramount with meatballs. To preview the flavor of yours, fry a bit of the meat mixture in a small pan and adjust as you go.

3. Make fat your friend
Meatballs should have the same level of fat as a burger—about 20 percent. To cut calories, use turkey breast, sirloin, or fish, but be sure not to overcook them.

4. Pick a partner
Sure, meatballs are great with spaghetti, but you can also pair them with soft polenta, mashed potatoes, or sticky rice, or stuff them inside a whole-wheat hoagie roll for a killer sandwich.

Garlic-Rosemary Roast Beef

Whatever happened to the days when the 6 p.m. dinner bell would ring and Mom would pull a beautifully browned roast from the oven? Well, plenty of things: microwaves, pizza delivery, the narrowing of the gender equality gap. Point is, we miss the roast, and there's no reason moms (and dads, brothers, and boyfriends!) shouldn't endeavor to make one every so often. It's as simple as turning on the oven, putting in the seasoned beef, and pulling it out when it's ready. This type of magic should be timeless.

You'll Need:

3 lb rump roast

8 cloves garlic, peeled and halved

2 Tbsp olive oil

½ Tbsp chopped fresh rosemary

Salt and black pepper to taste

How to Make It:

- Remove the roast from the fridge at least 30 minutes before cooking.

- Preheat the oven to 250°F. Use a small paring knife to make incisions into the roast and gently insert garlic clove halves all over. Rub the roast with the olive oil and season all over with the rosemary and plenty of salt and pepper. Place on a rack on a baking sheet and place in the middle rack of the oven.

- Roast for 90 minutes. Turn up the heat to 475°F and roast for another 15 minutes, until the beef has developed a deep-brown crust and an instant-read thermometer inserted in the thickest part registers 140°F.

Makes 6 to 8 servings

KITCHEN MACGYVER

No baking rack? No problem. Many recipes call for baking racks to allow the warm air to fully circulate around the meat, but you can simulate the effect very simply with no extra equipment. Position one oven rack in the middle of the oven and another immediately below it. Prep and season the meat, then place it directly on the middle rack. Place a rimmed baking sheet below to catch the juices as they fall from the meat. (Those precious juices can be turned into gravy with a bit of flour and broth!)

Per Serving

$2.09

260 calories

16 g fat
(5 g saturated)

380 mg sodium

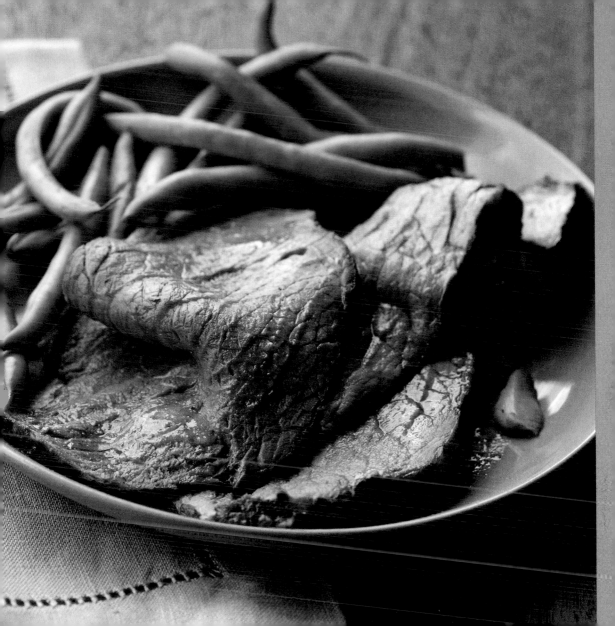

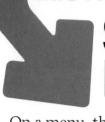

Eat This!

Smothered Pork Chops

On a menu, the word "smothered" foretells a certain type of nutritional doom, one dominated by butter (or worse, margarine or cheap oil) and cream, saturated fat and excess calories. At home, though, one can do all the smothering she wants and still walk away from the table feeling good about dinner. That's because in one's own kitchen, the smothering is done with a mixture of chicken stock, low-fat buttermilk, and sharp mustard, which combine with the cooking juices of the pork to create a beautiful—and low-calorie—blanket for the chop. Serve with Roasted Garlic Mashed Potatoes (page 302) and Honey-Roasted Carrots (page 316) for a perfect comfort feast.

You'll Need:

4 **thick center-cut pork chops (preferably bone-in), about 6 oz each**

Salt and black pepper to taste

Pinch of cayenne

1 **Tbsp butter**

2 **Tbsp flour**

1 **cup low-sodium chicken stock**

½ **cup low-fat buttermilk**

1 **tsp Dijon mustard**

Chopped fresh parsley for garnish (optional)

How to Make It:

● An hour before cooking, season the chops on both sides with salt, black pepper, and a bit of cayenne and return to the refrigerator. (You can skip this step, but it ensures a juicier, more fully seasoned chop.)

● Heat the butter in a large cast-iron skillet or sauté pan over medium heat. Dust the chops lightly with flour, coating both sides and shaking off any excess flour. Cook the chops, turning once, for 4 minutes per side, until nicely browned but not cooked all the way through. Remove to the cutting board.

● Add the stock, buttermilk, and mustard to the pan and simmer for 5 to 7 minutes, until the liquid is reduced by half. Return the chops to the pan and continue simmering for another 3 minutes or so, until they're just cooked through.

● Serve the chops with the gravy poured over the tops and garnished with a bit of parsley if using.

Makes 4 servings

Per Serving
$2.49
260 calories
15 g fat
(6 g saturated)
720 mg sodium

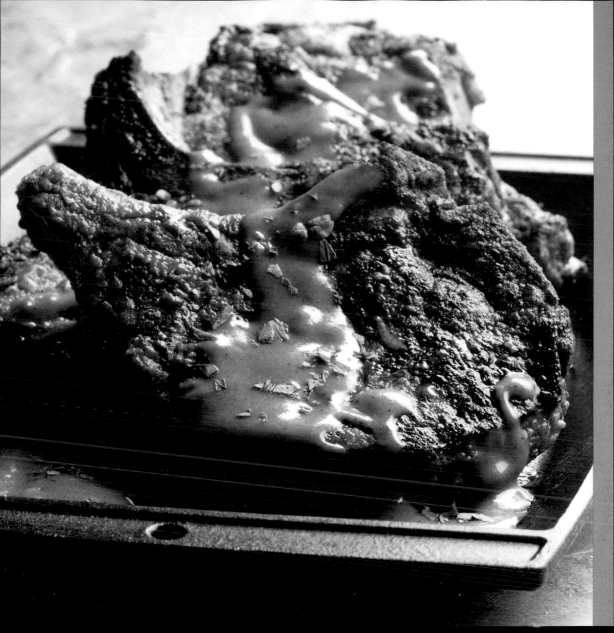

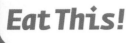

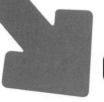

Crockpot Chili

Chili is particularly well suited to the slow cooker, since it's the type of dish that demands a long, slow simmer in order to seamlessly blend all the big flavors at play. And this chili has big flavors in spades: smoky chipotle pepper, hoppy IPA, and plenty of cumin and chili powder to tie the whole thing together. Chili and corn have a natural affinity for each other, so we like serving this with a wedge of cornbread or a stack of warm tortillas.

You'll Need:

- 1 Tbsp canola oil
- 2 lb chuck roast or sirloin tip, cut into ¾" cubes
- Salt and black pepper to taste
- 1 lb ground sirloin
- 1 large yellow onion, minced
- 3 cloves garlic, minced
- ¼ cup tomato paste
- 1 can or bottle (12 oz) IPA or stout
- 1 can (14 oz) crushed tomatoes
- 1 cup chicken broth
- 1 Tbsp chili powder (as good and freshly ground as you can get)
- 1 Tbsp chopped chipotle pepper
- 1 tsp cumin
- 2 bay leaves
- Pinch of cinnamon (optional)
- 1 can (14 oz) pinto beans
- Garnishes: chopped onion, chopped cilantro, sliced scallions, cubed avocado, pickled jalapeños, shredded Jack or Cheddar cheese

How to Make It:

- Heat the oil in a large cast-iron skillet or pan over medium-high heat. Season the cubes of chuck all over with salt and pepper. Working in batches, cook the chuck, turning occasionally, for 5 to 7 minutes, until nicely browned all over. Transfer to a slow cooker.

- In the same pan, cook the ground sirloin, onions, and garlic for about 10 minutes, until the sirloin is cooked through and the onions are soft. Stir in the tomato paste and beer, bring to a simmer, then pour it all over the beef in the slow cooker. Add the crushed tomatoes, broth, chili powder, chipotle, cumin, bay leaves, and cinnamon, if using. Set the slow cooker to high, cover, and cook for about 5 hours, until the chuck is fork-tender. Taste and season with more salt and black pepper if necessary. Stir in the pintos and cook until heated through. Discard the bay leaves and serve with your choice of garnishes.

Makes 10 servings

Per Serving
$1.80
250 calories
8 g fat
(2.5 g saturated)
500 mg sodium

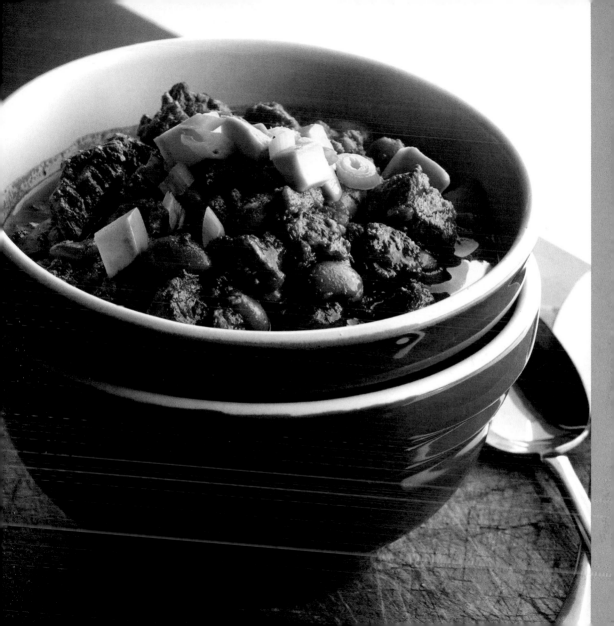

Eat This!

Bourbon-Glazed Ham with Peach Chutney

For most people, a baked ham is as rare a tabletop guest as a roast turkey—it's the kind of dish you're likely to see just once a year, around Christmastime. But unless you're brining and smoking your own (why would you, when amazing ready-to-cook hams await you at most supermarkets across the country?), ham's ease and overall awesomeness is tough to top. All you need to do is apply a glaze (in this case, a sweet-spicy mustard-bourbon sauce) and pop it in the oven for 45 minutes. And like that holiday turkey, the best thing about a baked ham is what's waiting for you in the fridge the next day.

You'll Need:

- ½ cup apricot or peach marmalade
- 2 Tbsp bourbon
- 2 Tbsp Dijon mustard
- Black pepper to taste
- 1 (9-pound) bone-in smoked ham (such as Smithfield)
- 3 peaches, pitted, peeled, and chopped
- ½ small red onion, diced
- 1 clove garlic, minced
- 1 jalapeño pepper, minced
- 1 cup orange juice
- 1 Tbsp apple cider vinegar

How to Make It:

- Preheat the oven to 400°F.
- Combine the marmalade, bourbon, mustard, and plenty of black pepper in a mixing bowl. Use a knife to score the skin side of the ham, cutting 1 inch down into the meat to create diamonds. Spread the glaze all over the ham, rubbing into the cracks created by the scoring. Place on the middle rack of the oven and bake for 45 minutes, until the glaze caramelizes and browns on the surface of the ham.
- While the ham cooks, make the chutney: Combine the peaches, onion, garlic, jalapeño, juice, and vinegar in a saucepan over medium heat. Bring to a boil, then turn the heat down just enough to maintain a bare simmer. Cook for about 15 minutes, until the fruit is soft and most of the liquid has evaporated.
- Slice the ham and serve with the chutney.

Makes 16 servings

Per Serving
$1.97
350 calories
11 g fat
(5 g saturated)
920 mg sodium

LEFTOVER♥LOVE

Both the meat and the bone, suffused with smoky intensity, contain incredible next-day potential. Here are a few of our favorites.

- Scrambled eggs with ham, scallion, and sharp Cheddar
- Ham, arugula, and peach marmalade sandwich
- Baby spinach salad with ham, dried cranberries, pumpkin seeds, and goat cheese
- Split Pea Soup (page 108), the perfect follow-up to this dinner

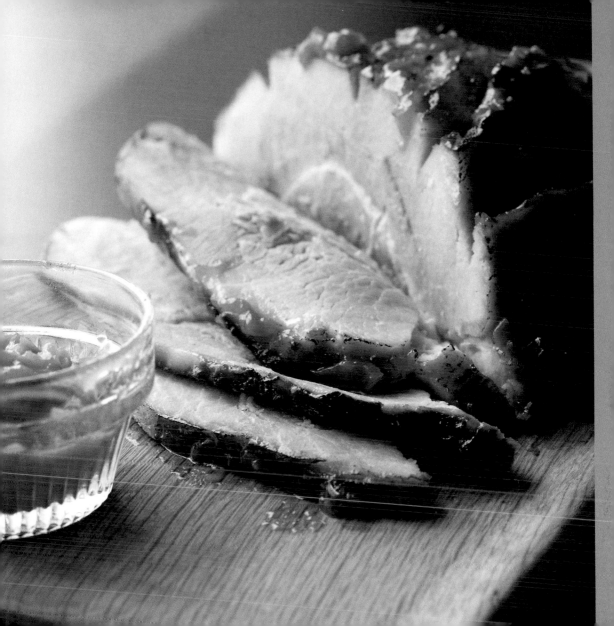

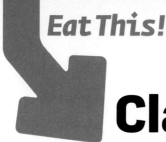

Classic Beef Stew

It's the dead of winter. You've endured a long day of injustices at the office and you arrive home cold, wet, famished. But when you open the front door the smell hits you: beef and red wine and vegetables, slow-cooked into a state of deliciousness while you worked. Now that's comfort.

You'll Need:

- 1 Tbsp canola oil
- 3 lb sirloin roast, brisket, or chuck, cut into 1" cubes
- 1 Tbsp flour
- Salt and black pepper to taste
- 2 medium onions, chopped
- 1 cup dry red wine, such as Pinot Noir or Cabernet Sauvignon
- 2 Tbsp tomato paste
- 2 cups chicken broth
- 3 bay leaves
- 8 branches fresh thyme (or 1 tsp dried)
- 6 medium red potatoes, cut into ½" pieces
- 3 medium carrots, peeled and chopped
- 2 cups frozen pearl onions
- 1 cup frozen peas
- Chopped fresh parsley or gremolata (optional; see note)

How to Make It:

- Heat ½ tablespoon of the oil in a large cast-iron skillet or sauté pan over medium-high heat. Combine the beef and flour in a bowl, season with salt and pepper, and toss to lightly coat the beef. Working in two batches to avoid crowding the pan, sear the beef in the hot oil, turning occasionally, until nicely browned. Transfer to a slow cooker.

- Add the remaining oil to the skillet. Add the chopped onions and cook for about 5 minutes, until lightly browned. Stir in the wine and tomato paste, scraping the bottom of the pan to free up any browned bits. Pour the onion mixture over the beef, then add the broth, bay leaves, and thyme. Set the slow cooker to high, cover, and cook for about 4 hours (or on low for 8 hours), until the beef is fork-tender.

- An hour before serving, add the potatoes, carrots, and pearl onions. Five minutes before serving, add the peas. Discard the bay leaves and thyme branches and season with salt and black pepper. Serve garnished with parsley or gremolata if you like.

Makes 8 servings

Per Serving

$2.56

410 calories
13 g fat
(4 g saturated)
600 mg sodium

SECRET WEAPON

Gremolata

While classic beef stew comes with no splashy garnishes, intense meaty dishes like this one are best when finished with a fresh, contrasting note. Cue gremolata, a combination of garlic, parsley, and lemon used to garnish bold Italian dishes like osso buco. The combination also works perfectly on top of grilled steak, roast chicken, and even pasta. To make, combine 2 tablespoons minced garlic with ½ cup minced fresh parsley and 1 tablespoon grated lemon zest.

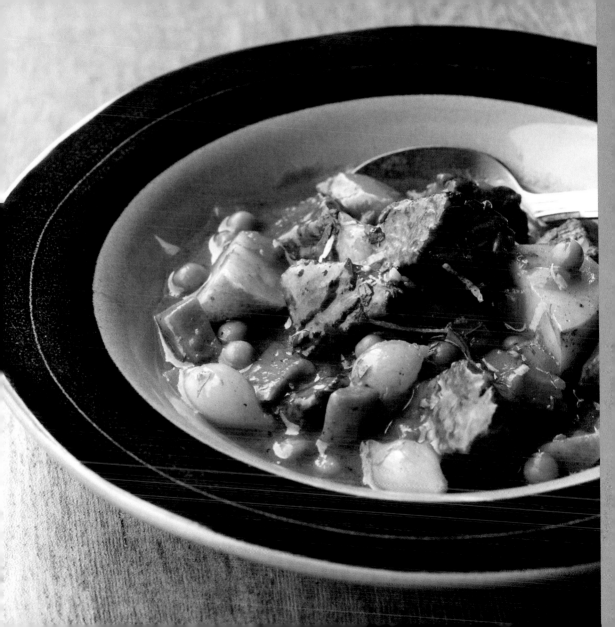

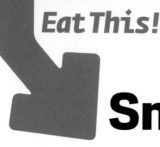
Smoky Ribs with Peach BBQ Sauce

Pit masters can spend 10 hours feeding their smokers to sweat out a few racks of ribs. We admire the dedication, but when it comes to home cooking, there's an easier way to make amazing ribs. It starts in the oven, where spice-rubbed ribs are slow-roasted until tender. From there they go to the grill for a concentrated blast of hickory smoke. Finish with a barbecue sauce spiked with bourbon and peach and you have ribs any barbecue baron could respect.

You'll Need:

- 2 medium racks baby back ribs
- ½ Tbsp chili powder
- 1 Tbsp brown sugar
- Salt and black pepper to taste
- ½ cup Classic Barbecue Sauce (page 319) or favorite barbecue sauce
- 2 Tbsp bourbon (optional)
- 1 very ripe peach, peeled and pitted
- 2 cups hickory chips, soaked in water for 30 minutes

How to Make It:

- Preheat the oven to 300°F. Rub the top sides of the ribs with the chili powder and brown sugar and season with salt and black pepper. Place the racks on a baking sheet, cover with foil, and bake for 90 minutes, until the meat is tender but not falling completely off the bone.

- While the ribs cook, combine the barbecue sauce, bourbon (if using), and peach in a food processor or blender and puree.

- Preheat a grill over medium heat. Place the chips in a wood-chip box (or in a foil packet, see "Kitchen MacGyver," right) and place the box below the grill grate, directly over the flame (if using charcoal, sprinkle the chips directly over the fire). Place the ribs on the grill, close the lid, and allow the meat to absorb the smoke for 15 to 20 minutes. Paint the ribs with a generous amount of the barbecue sauce. Close the lid and continue cooking for another 15 minutes, until the sauce caramelizes on the ribs.

- Remove the ribs and brush once more with the sauce before serving.

Makes 6 to 8 servings

Per Serving
$2.76
410 calories
31 g fat
(11 g saturated)
460 mg sodium

KITCHEN MACGYVER

A full-blown smoker is out of the question for most people, but that doesn't mean you can't achieve the smoky effect with your current setup. A wood-chip box holds the chips directly above a gas or charcoal fire as the heat releases their aroma. Failing that, you can make a wood-chip packet with a large piece of aluminum foil—just be sure to poke holes in it so that the smoke can escape. In either case, soak the wood chips before adding to the fire; damp chips will smoke more than dry ones.

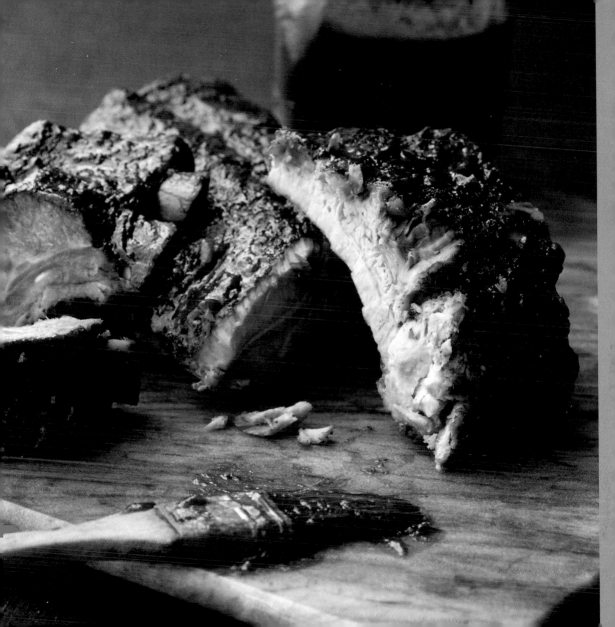

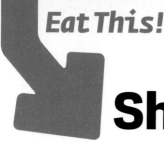

Eat This!

Shepherd's Pie

Like so many of the world's great comfort foods, shepherd's pie was born of humble origins, invented as a way of using up old scraps of meat, with the vegetables and the potato topping used to stretch the dish into extra portions. This is meat-and-potato fare at its finest: a slow-simmered mixture of ground red meat and vegetables blanketed with a warm cover of mashed potatoes. The dish is traditionally made with lamb (you know, since shepherds look after sheep), but sirloin makes a leaner and perfectly tasty pie.

You'll Need:

- 2 medium russet potatoes, peeled and cubed
- Salt and black pepper to taste
- 2 Tbsp butter
- ¾ cup 2% milk
- ½ Tbsp olive oil
- 1 medium onion, diced
- 3 medium carrots, peeled and diced
- 2 cloves garlic, minced
- 1 lb ground sirloin or ground lamb
- 1 Tbsp flour
- 2 Tbsp tomato paste
- 1 cup low-sodium beef stock
- 1 tsp Worcestershire
- 1 tsp chopped fresh rosemary
- 1 cup frozen peas

Per Serving
$2.76
380 calories
14 g fat
(6 g saturated)
510 mg sodium

How to Make It:

- Preheat the oven to 400°F.
- Place the potatoes in a medium saucepan, cover with water, and season with a pinch of salt. Cook for about 15 minutes, until the potatoes are tender all the way through. Press through a potato ricer (if you have one) or mash with a masher or a pair of forks. Stir in the butter and milk and season with salt and black pepper.
- Meanwhile, heat the olive oil in a large sauté pan over medium heat. Add the onions, carrots, and garlic and cook for about 5 minutes, until soft. Add the ground meat and cook for about 5 minutes, until no longer pink. Stir in the flour and tomato sauce and stir so that the ingredients are evenly coated. Add the stock, Worcestershire, and rosemary and simmer for 15 minutes. Add the peas and season with salt and black pepper.
- Pour the meat and vegetable mixture into a 13" x 9" baking dish and spread into an even layer. Top with the mashed potatoes. Bake for about 25 minutes, until the potatoes are nicely browned on the surface.

Makes 4 servings

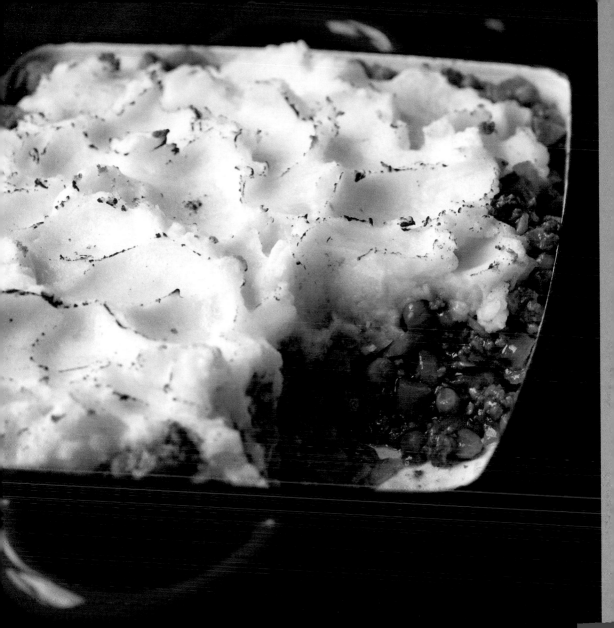

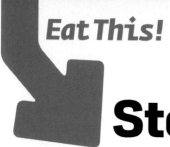

Steaks with Red Wine Sauce

Beyond mere convenience, cooking a steak indoors offers a few huge benefits over outdoor grilling: It's easier to control the temperature of the stovetop, which means it's easier to create a crust on the outside and a rosy warm center within. Plus the pan captures those vital bits of browned meat and escaped juices, which form the base for a rich sauce to pour over the steak. It's the kind of simple technique that makes you look like a pro in the kitchen.

You'll Need:

- ½ Tbsp olive oil
- 2 (12 oz each) sirloin, skirt, or flank steaks

Salt and black pepper to taste

- 1 medium shallot, minced
- 1 cup red wine
- 1 cup beef broth
- 2 Tbsp cold butter, cut into small pieces
- 1 Tbsp fresh thyme leaves or 2 Tbsp chopped parsley

How to Make It:

- Heat the olive oil in a large cast-iron skillet or stainless-steel pan over medium-high heat. Season the steaks on both sides with salt and plenty of black pepper. When the oil is lightly smoking, add the steaks to the pan. Cook, turning every minute or so, for about 8 minutes total, until the steaks are deeply browned and firm but yielding to the touch. Remove to a cutting board to rest.

- Add the shallot to the same pan and sauté for 1 minute, until softened. Pour in the red wine and the broth, scraping the bottom of the pan to release any brown bits. Cook over high heat for 5 minutes, until the liquid is reduced by three-quarters. Remove from the heat and whisk in the butter one piece at a time. Stir in the parsley.

- Slice the steaks into thick pieces, arrange on 4 warm plates, and pour the red wine sauce over the pieces.

Makes 4 servings

Per Serving
$3.92
380 calories
18 g fat
(6 g saturated)
410 mg sodium

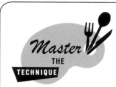

Master THE **TECHNIQUE**

Pan Sauce

Steak makes for the most classic pan sauce, but the technique can be used for other meats and fish as well. Follow the steps in the recipe (remove protein, add aromatics and liquid, scrape pan, reduce liquid, stir in cold butter) for any of these combinations:

- **CHICKEN BREASTS OR THIGHS:** garlic, sherry or port, chicken broth, rosemary

- **PORK CHOPS:** garlic, ginger, orange juice, soy sauce

- **FIRM WHITE FISH:** fresh thyme or parsley, white wine, lemon juice

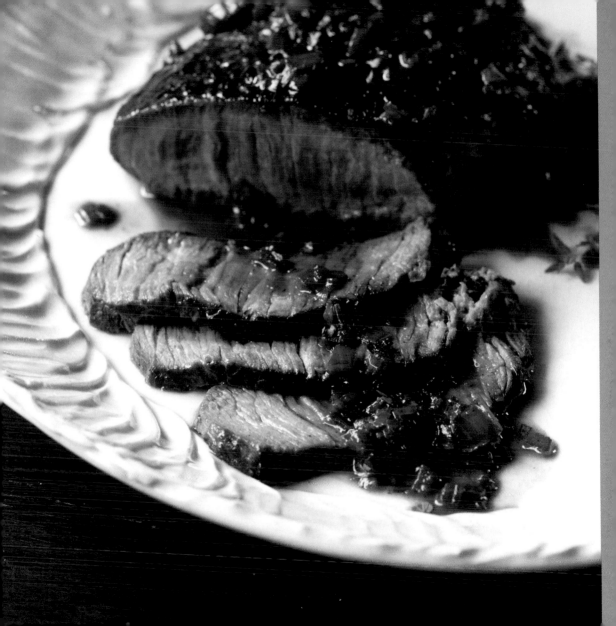

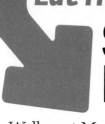

Eat This!

Slow-Roasted Pork Shoulder

Walk past Momofuku Ssäm Bar in New York's East Village any night around 8 p.m. and you'll see a table of eight or so lucky diners, jaws agape, tucking into a heroic hunk of pork just like this. It's a dramatic dish, one that you want to bring to a table crowded with ravenous friends and loved ones. You can serve the pork with a variety of amazing accoutrements—from salsa and guac and corn tortillas for tacos, to lettuce leaves and Asian condiments for Korean-style wraps (as it's served at Ssäm Bar). But, truthfully, it's delicious enough to be dinner on its own.

You'll Need:

- 1 **(6 to 8 lb) boneless pork shoulder**
- 2 **Tbsp salt**
- ¼ **cup granulated sugar**
- ½ **cup brown sugar**

How to Make It:

- The night before cooking, rub the pork all over with the salt and the granulated sugar. Cover and return to the refrigerator to brine overnight.
- Preheat the oven to 300°F. Place the pork in a large baking dish and roast on the bottom rack, using a baster or a large spoon to baste the pork every 30 minutes or so. (If you want to leave the pork in the oven and forget about it, it will still come out great without basting.) The pork is done when it easily pulls apart with a fork, about 5 hours.
- Remove the pork from the oven and increase the oven temperature to 475°F. Rub the pork all over with the brown sugar and return to the oven. Roast for about 15 minutes, until the sugar forms a dark mahogany crust. Serve as is with a few vegetable sides, or in any of the manners outlined in "Meal Multiplier," right.

Makes 12 to 16 servings

Per Serving
$1.96
410 calories
22 g fat
(8 g saturated)
900 mg sodium

MEAL MULTIPLIER

This fork-tender mountain of pork can be the star of a dozen different final dishes. Here are just a few sources of inspiration:

- **MEXICAN:** Corn tortillas, black beans, salsa, guacamole
- **KOREAN:** Bibb lettuce leaves, steamed rice, hoisin, sriracha
- **CAROLINA:** Apple cider vinegar spiked with chili flakes, cole slaw, potato rolls

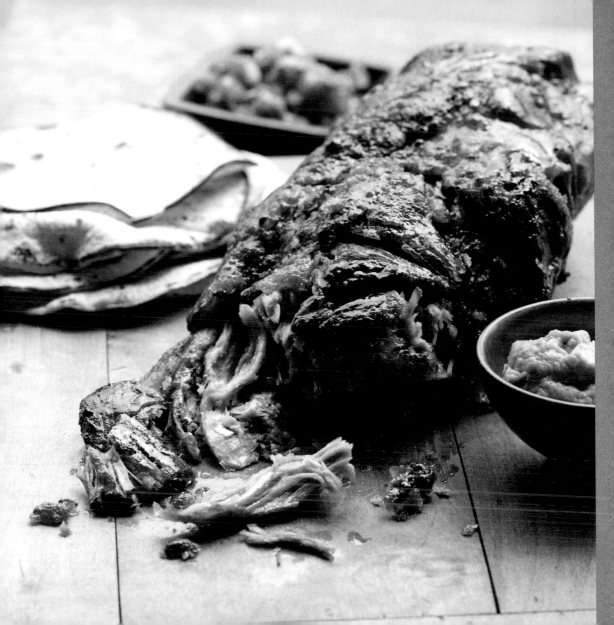

Carne Asada Burritos

The modern burrito is a tortilla swollen to the size of Chuck Norris's bicep, stuffed to the point of bursting with meat, cheese, and condiments. Delicious stuff, but capable of packing up to 1,500 calories a pop. Our version, modestly scaled down, concentrates on the most important parts of the burrito: guac, black beans, and, above all, juicy chunks of marinated skirt steak.

You'll Need:

- ½ cup orange juice
- 2 Tbsp canola or vegetable oil
- 1 Tbsp chipotle pepper purée
- 1 tsp cumin
- 4 cloves garlic
- 1 lb skirt or flank steak
- Salt and black pepper to taste
- 4 large whole-wheat tortillas
- ½ cup shredded Jack cheese
- 4 Tbsp Guacamole (page 320), or high-quality packaged guacamole like Wholly Guacamole
- 1 cup Pico de Gallo (page 319)
- 1 can (15 oz) black or pinto beans, drained

How to Make It:

- Combine the juice, oil, chipotle purée, cumin, and garlic in a blender and puree. Place the steak in a sealable plastic bag and cover with the marinade. Marinate in the refrigerator for at least 1 hour or up to 8 hours.

- Preheat a grill over high heat. Remove the steak from the marinade, pat dry with paper towels, and season all over with salt and black pepper. Grill, turning occasionally, for 8 minutes, until the surface is nicely browned and the meat is firm but still yielding to the touch. Remove and rest for at least 5 minutes before chopping into bite-size pieces.

- Heat a cast-iron skillet or nonstick pan over low heat. Place a tortilla in the center and warm on one side for 30 seconds. Flip and cover with 2 tablespoons of the cheese. Continue heating until gently toasted. Remove to a plate and top with 1 tablespoon guacamole, ¼ cup pico de gallo, and one-quarter of the beans and steak. Fold opposite sides over toward the center, then roll the tortilla to create a tight, sealed burrito. Repeat with the remaining tortillas.

Makes 4 servings

Per Serving
$3.37
420 calories
20 g fat
(6 g saturated)
660 mg sodium

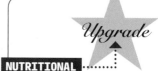

Upgrade

NUTRITIONAL

Burritos are fine every so often, but you can achieve the same harmony of flavors by making tacos instead. Follow the same marinated steak recipe, but ditch the big tortilla and serve the meat with a pile of lightly grilled corn tortillas instead—plus all of the fixings, of course. A pile of grilled scallions, a staple of taco carts all over Mexico, makes for a nice side dish.

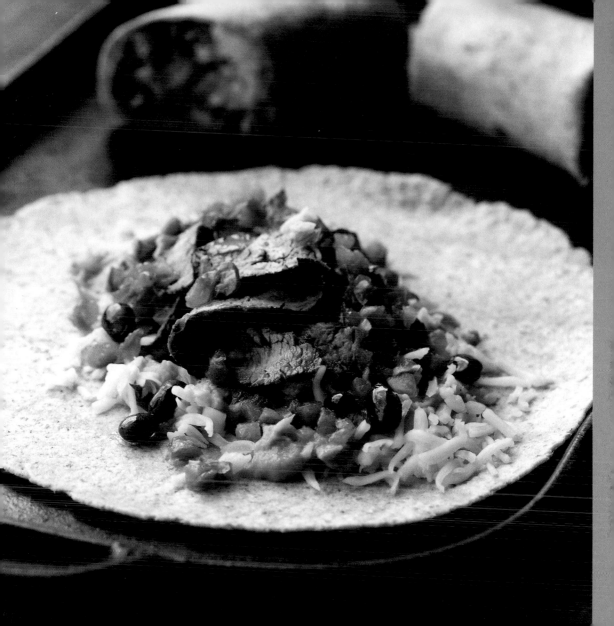

Poor Man's Steak with Garlicky Gravy

This country has fallen on lean times in recent years, but unfortunately the figurative belt-tightening doesn't seem to be accompanied by a literal one. That's because the most potent sources of calories and seasoning (oil, sugar, salt) are still cheap and more common in restaurant cooking than ever. Here, we fuse health, flavor, and affordability in a way only good home cooking can. Inexpensive lean ground sirloin is formed into steaks, then covered with mushrooms, onions, and a soy-spiked sauce good enough to make your doormat taste delicious. Serve this decadent mess over a bed of mashed potatoes, or for a healthier, easier sidekick, Garlic-Lemon Spinach (page 312).

You'll Need:

- 1 lb ground sirloin or chuck, shaped into 4 equal patties
- 1½ Tbsp canola oil, divided
- Salt and ground black pepper to taste
- 2 cloves garlic, minced
- 1 yellow onion, sliced
- 4 oz white or cremini mushrooms, stems removed, sliced
- ½ Tbsp flour
- ½ cup beef or chicken stock
- 1 Tbsp ketchup
- 1 Tbsp low-sodium soy sauce
- 1 tsp Worcestershire sauce

How to Make It:

- Preheat the oven to 200°F.
- Heat a large cast-iron skillet or sauté pan over medium-high heat.
- Season the patties all over with salt and pepper. Add 1 Tbsp oil to the pan and cook until a nicely browned crust forms on the patties, about 3 to 4 minutes, then flip and continue cooking for another 3 to 4 minutes for medium-rare. Move the patties to a baking sheet and place in the oven to keep warm.
- Add the remaining oil and the garlic, onions, and mushrooms to the same pan, and cook until the vegetables begin to brown nicely, about 5 to 7 minutes. Sprinkle the flour over the vegetables, stir so that it coats them evenly, then add the stock, using a whisk to keep lumps from forming. Stir in the ketchup, soy sauce, and Worcestershire sauce and continue cooking until the gravy thickens, another 2 to 3 minutes. Serve the patties on a bed of mashed potatoes or sautéed spinach (or both) with the gravy drizzled over the top.

Makes 4 servings

Per Serving
$1.81
220 calories
9 g fat
(3 g saturated)
470 mg sodium

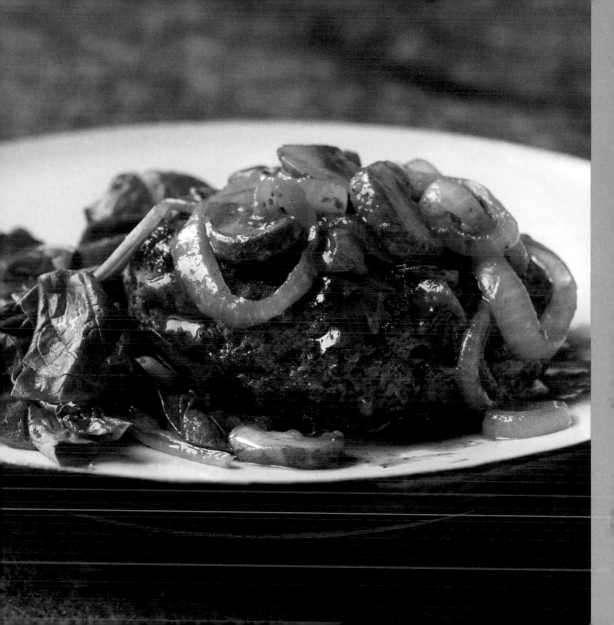

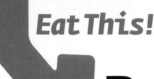

Braised Brisket
with Horseradish Cream

Brisket is a notoriously tough piece of meat. It takes the best pit masters up to 18 hours of low-temperature smoking to wrestle the beef into a state of acceptable tenderness. But through the miracle of the slow cooker, where moisture and heat combine to turn even the toughest cuts into spoon-tender masterpieces, brisket can be worked into a state of soul-soothing deliciousness with only about 15 minutes of prep work.

You'll Need:

- 1 Tbsp olive oil
- 3 lb brisket (preferably with a thin fat cap still attached)
- Salt and black pepper to taste
- 1 bottle (12 oz) dark beer
- 2 cups low-sodium chicken stock
- 2 Tbsp tomato paste
- 2 large yellow onions, quartered
- 1 bunch carrots, peeled
- 8 cloves garlic, peeled
- 2 bay leaves
- ¼ cup 2% Greek yogurt
- 2 Tbsp chopped fresh parsley
- 1 Tbsp prepared horseradish

How to Make It:

- Heat the olive oil in a large cast-iron skillet or sauté pan. Season the brisket all over with salt and black pepper. Sear in the pan for about 7 minutes, until all sides are nicely browned. Place in a slow cooker. Add the beer to the pan and scrape up any browned bits. Pour over the brisket. Add the stock, tomato paste, onions, carrots, garlic, and bay leaves to the slow cooker. Cover and cook on high for 4 hours (or on low for up to 8 hours), until the brisket is very tender.

- Combine the yogurt, parsley, and horseradish in a mixing bowl.

- Remove the brisket from the cooker and slice into thin pieces. Discard the bay leaves. Serve the brisket in a shallow, wide bowl with the onions, carrots, and a bit of broth poured over the top. Garnish each serving with a scoop of the horseradish cream.

Makes 10 servings

Per Serving
$2.47
380 calories
25 g fat
(8 g saturated)
350 mg sodium

LEFTOVER♥LOVE

Three ways to turn extra brisket into a next-day bounty:

- **BRISKET FRENCH DIP:** Slice the brisket thinly, top with caramelized onions and Swiss. Serve with a warm cup of the braising liquid.

- **CORNED BEEF HASH:** Cook diced potatoes and onions in a pan until soft, then stir in shredded brisket, Dijon mustard, Worcestershire, and some of the leftover braising liquid.

- **BRISKET NACHOS:** Shred the meat, then use it to top tortilla chips along with pepper-Jack cheese, pinto beans, sliced jalapeños, and salsa verde.

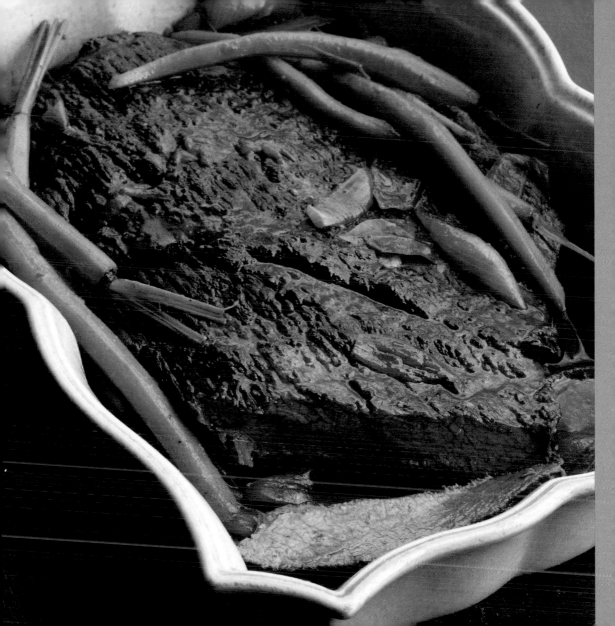

CHAPTER 9

SEAFOOD

America's Worst FISH

Perkins's Jumbo Shrimp Dinner with French Fries and Broccoli

1,240 calories
69 g fat
(18 g saturated)
2,610 mg sodium
Price: $9.99

Shrimp plates are one of the few restaurant dishes that consistently fall on either extreme of the health spectrum, and there's usually only one factor determining the crustacean's nutritional fate: the deep fryer. Order your shrimp grilled or sautéed, and you reap the benefits of the seafood's lean protein. Opt for fried fish, and you may as well be eating a cheeseburger. And while we're on the topic of the detrimental effects of fried fare, since when did french fries become a suitable seafood side?

Eat This Instead!
Shrimp & Grits (page 252)

340 calories
10 g fat
(4 g saturated)
610 mg sodium
Cost per serving: $3.24
Save! 900 calories and $6.75!

Cheesecake Factory's Shrimp and Chicken Gumbo

1,570 calories
N/A g fat
(37 g saturated fat)
2,249 mg sodium
Price: $16.95

Depending on the recipe, gumbo can run the gamut from lean and light to heavy and salty. The traditional Cajun version is usually thickened with flour and butter, and—not one to shy away from fattening fare—the Cheesecake Factory sticks to tradition.

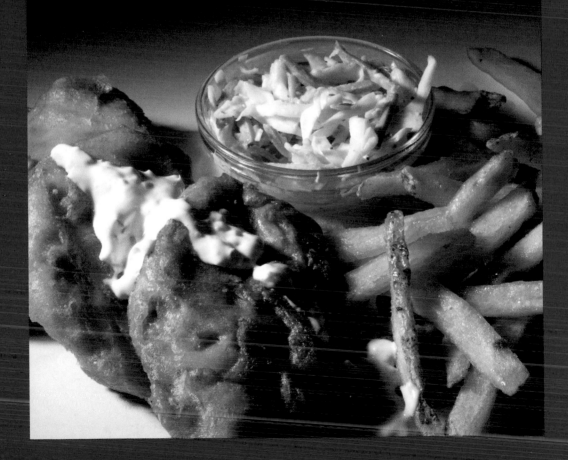

1,930 calories

A plate as beige as Applebee's fish and chips can never be a good thing.

But it takes more than a scoop of flour and a stick of butter to reach the Factory's signature sky-high calorie counts; the rest of the calories in this New Orleans classic come from a mountain of refined white rice in the center of the bowl. Cioppino provides the same deep, slow-simmered flavor of gumbo, but forgoes nearly 2 days' worth of saturated fat for a huge helping of heart-healthy omega-3 fatty acids.

Eat This Instead!
Cioppino (page 246)
280 calories
6 g fat (1 g saturated)
760 mg sodium
Cost per serving: $4.50
Save! 1,290 calories and $12.45!

WORST FISH TACOS
On The Border's Dos XX Fish Tacos with Creamy Red Chile Sauce (without rice)
1,670 calories
116 g fat (27 g saturated)
2,910 mg sodium
Price: $9.99

We don't always eat tacos, but when we do, we certainly don't eat Dos XX. A deep-fried battering, a cream-sauce smothering, and a flour-tortilla flogging leave this fish dish with as many calories as 10 Taco Bell Crunchy Tacos. Sure, there are other fish in the sea, but if you want a serious seafood dinner, make it at home. We pair the spice of blackened tilapia with the cool of lime butter. Wrap it

all in a warm corn tortilla with a bit of salsa and you have yourself The World's Most Interesting Fish Taco.

Eat This Instead!
Blackened Tilapia with Garlic-Lime Butter (page 248)
300 calories
14 g fat (6 g saturated)
510 mg sodium
Cost per serving: $2.32
Save! 1,370 calories and $7.67!

WORST SALMON
Cheesecake Factory's Miso Salmon
1,740 calories
N/A g fat (40 g saturated)
2,354 mg sodium
Price: $19.95

We feel bad for this fish's PR team. What could be more scandalous than a plate of salmon—the epitome of a healthy protein—saddled with 2 days' worth of saturated fat and close to a day's calories? What's worse, this dish is one of the most disturbing health-food frauds we've found. The side of snow peas and the glaze of soybean-based miso are usually nutritional no-brainers, and the scoop of white rice—while not particularly healthy—certainly doesn't pack the caloric punch to deliver such a massive blow to your diet. Guess that's what you get when you let straitlaced salmon hang out with the ruffians in the restaurant world.

Eat This Instead!
Roast Salmon with Lentils (page 250)
440 calories
12 g fat (2 g saturated)
680 mg sodium
Cost per serving: $3.35
Save! 1,300 calories and $16.60!

WORST FISH AND CHIPS
Applebee's New England Fish and Chips
1,930 calories
138 g fat
(24 g saturated, 1.5 g trans)
3,180 mg sodium
Price: $9.99

We've said it before, and we'll say it again: When fish hits the fryer, your diet hits the skids. At chains like Applebee's, a dousing of hot oil can result in a seafood selection with nearly a day's calories, plus when you venture too far from shore—and by shore, we mean your kitchen—you run the risk of encountering treacherous waves of trans fatty acids. The fish plate here packs close to the maximum recommended intake of trans fats, which is surprising considering Applebee's swore off the heart-hurting nutrient in 2007. Fishy.

Eat This Instead!
Fish and Chips (page 240)
380 calories
14 g fat (1.5 g saturated)
810 mg sodium
Cost per serving: $4.29
Save! 1,550 calories and $5.70!

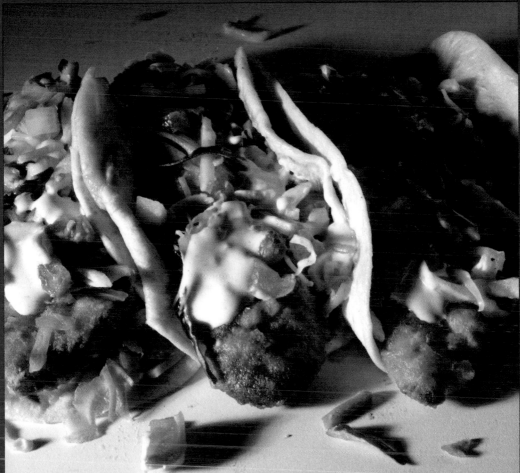

116 grams of fat

On the Border makes the fishiest tacos we've ever seen.

8-Inch Plates

We're living in a super-sized world. We drive to work in tank-like SUVs, buy our groceries in warehouse-sized supermarkets, and return home to double-decker houses with spare bedrooms and two-car garages. Our television screens fill entire walls. And yes, not surprisingly, our portions and even our serving vessels have gotten bigger and bigger along the way.

According to a *Journal of Consumer Research* study published earlier this year, the average dinner plate has increased 23 percent, from 9.6 inches to 11.8 inches, since the early 20th century. That same study found that when eating off larger plates, people underestimate serving sizes—a finding that only reinforces numerous other studies showing that appetite is largely dependent on environmental cues.

This calls up one of the big challenges of eating reasonably: When you're eating off a manhole-sized dinner plate, a modest scoop of spaghetti looks almost comical—like a kid wearing his father's suit jacket. So you add a couple more scoops, and go about cleaning your plate. You've just super-sized your meal, tripled your caloric intake, and undermined your best efforts to lose weight. The worst part: The food wasn't any better, richer, or more delicious. There was just, well, a lot more of it.

Thankfully, the fix for this silent weight-gain culprit is as easy as stocking your cabinet with a new set of plates.

OUR PICK

BASIC WHITE 8-INCH SALAD PLATES
$15.99 for set of 8 Target.com

Today's "salad" plate was once considered adequate for dinner—and it still is. Use these smaller plates in place of your usual 10- or 12-inch plates and you'll soon find that your jeans are fitting a little looser.

Small Plate
SUPERPOWERS

DOWNSIZE DINNER

In recent years, researchers at the Cornell Food and Brand Lab have discovered a lot about how serving dishes affect how much we consume. The takeaway is this: Use smaller plates because you'll be less likely to overeat if you keep the plates and bowls small.

Worried the small plate won't provide enough food to fill your stomach? Don't be. Looking at an empty plate makes your brain more likely to fire off a fullness signal, so while you can always go back for seconds, there's a good chance you won't want to.

CUT CALORIES WITH COLOR

Another finding from the *Journal of Consumer Research* study was that people feel like they're eating more food when the plate-to-food color contrast is highest. So red plates accentuate green foods, purple plates accentuate yellow foods, and so on. To maximize color contrast with as many recipes as possible, keep a set of 8-inch white plates in your cabinet (white provides the most universally high-contrast backdrop) plus have a handful of other primary color plates on hand to contrast your more colorful creations.

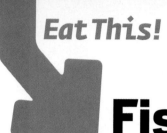

Fish & Chips

We love everything about the idea of fish and chips—the crunch of the batter playing off the tender bite of the fish, the pile of crispy potatoes, the dollop of tartar sauce or splash of malt vinegar served on the side. This playful ode to the English staple combines all of the fish and chips experience in one bite, using crushed salt and vinegar potato chips to coat cod fillets, which are then baked until crispy and golden brown. The only thing it leaves out of the equation is the most regrettable part of fish and chips: all those excess calories from the deep fryer. If you want real chips on the side, we suggest Crispy Oven-Baked Fries (page 298) or Smoked Paprika Potato Chips (page 317).

You'll Need:

- 4 cod fillets, 6 oz each
- 1 cup nonfat buttermilk

Tabasco to taste

- ¾ cup panko bread crumbs
- ¾ cup crushed salt and vinegar chips

Salt and black pepper to taste

- 2 Tbsp olive oil mayonnaise
- 2 Tbsp Greek yogurt

Juice of 1 lemon

- 2 Tbsp chopped pickles
- 1 Tbsp capers
- 1 tsp Dijon mustard

How to Make It:

- Combine the cod, buttermilk, and a few shakes of Tabasco in a sealable plastic bag. Marinate in the refrigerator for 20 minutes.

- Preheat the oven to 400°F. Combine the bread crumbs and crushed chips in a shallow baking dish and season with a few pinches of salt and black pepper. Working with one piece at a time, remove the fish from the buttermilk and roll in the coating, using your fingers to pat the mixture onto the surface of the fish.

- Place the coated fish onto a rack set in a baking sheet. Bake for about 15 minutes, until the coating is nicely browned and crunchy and the fish flakes with gentle pressure from your finger.

- While the fish bakes, combine the mayo, yogurt, lemon juice, pickles, capers, and Dijon in a mixing bowl. Serve the fish with a scoop of tartar sauce on the side.

Makes 4 servings

Per Serving
$4.29
380 calories
14 g fat
(1.5 g saturated)
810 mg sodium

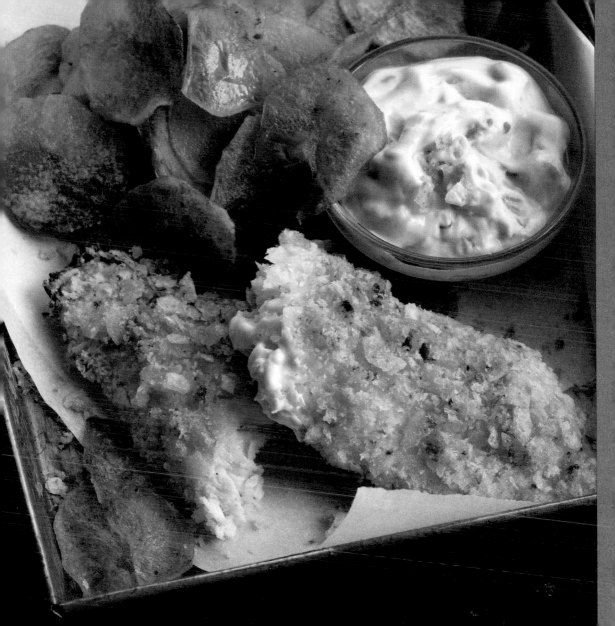

Spanish Garlic Shrimp

A staple on Spanish tapas menus everywhere, *gambas al ajillo* is a dead simple but genius combination of shrimp slow-cooked in olive oil that's been infused with lots of garlic, smoked paprika, and a touch of chile heat. Serve it as an appetizer and everyone will beg you for the recipe. Serve it with a scoop of couscous and some roasted asparagus, and you have a magical weeknight dinner. Either way, you'll need a bit of bread to drag through the garlicky olive oil at the bottom of the pot.

You'll Need:

- ¼ cup olive oil
- 6 cloves garlic, thinly sliced
- ¼ tsp red pepper flakes
- 1 lb medium shrimp, peeled and deveined
- ½ tsp smoked paprika

Salt to taste

- ¼ cup chopped fresh parsley

How to Make It:

- Combine the olive oil, garlic, and red pepper in a medium sauté pan set over very low heat. Cook slowly for about 5 minutes, until very soft and caramelized, being careful not to let it burn.
- Season the shrimp with the smoked paprika and salt and add to the pan. Sauté, turning once, for about 4 minutes total, just until cooked through. Sprinkle in the parsley and serve with bread for dunking into the garlic oil.

Makes 4 servings

Per Serving
$2.65
250 calories
15 g fat
(2 g saturated)
310 mg sodium

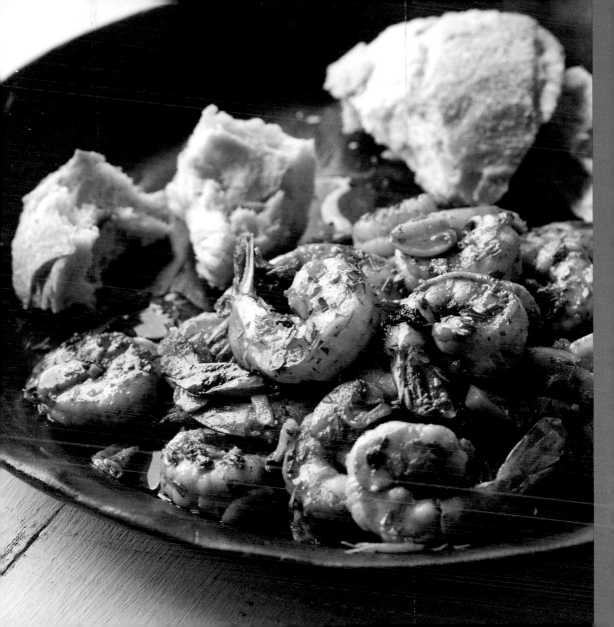

Cornmeal Catfish with Tomato Gravy

The idea for this recipe comes from one of the kings of comfort food, Sean Brock, who cooks up soul-rattling Southern dishes at his Charleston restaurant, Husk. Sean has an incredible gift for making food you will crave months after eating: crispy chicken skins with peach marmalade, shrimp and grits with charred peppers, fried green tomatoes topped with pimento cheese and country ham. But what haunts us the most is his catfish with a simple tomato gravy, a recipe from that endless source of comfort food the world over, a grandmother—Sean's, to be precise.

You'll Need:

- 2 Tbsp rendered bacon fat
- 2 Tbsp plus ½ cup ground cornmeal
- 1 can (14.5 oz) whole peeled tomatoes, lightly crushed, juices discarded

Salt and black pepper to taste

- 1 Tbsp canola oil
- ⅛ tsp cayenne pepper
- 4 catfish fillets (about 6 oz each)

How to Make It:

- Heat the bacon fat in a medium saucepan over low heat. Add the 2 tablespoons cornmeal and continue cooking, stirring constantly, for about 5 minutes, until the cornmeal is light brown. Add the drained tomatoes and simmer for another 10 minutes. Season with salt and black pepper.

- While the sauce simmers, prepare the catfish: Heat the oil in a large cast-iron skillet or nonstick pan over medium heat. Spread the ½ cup of cornmeal out in a shallow dish and season with the cayenne, plus a few good pinches of salt and black pepper. Dust the catfish on both sides with the cornmeal and place in the hot pan. Cook, turning once, for 6 to 8 minutes, until the surface is golden brown and crusty and the fish flakes with gentle pressure from your finger. Serve each fillet with a big scoop of tomato gravy.

Makes 4 servings

Per Serving
$2.67
340 calories
16 g fat
(3.5 g saturated)
500 mg sodium

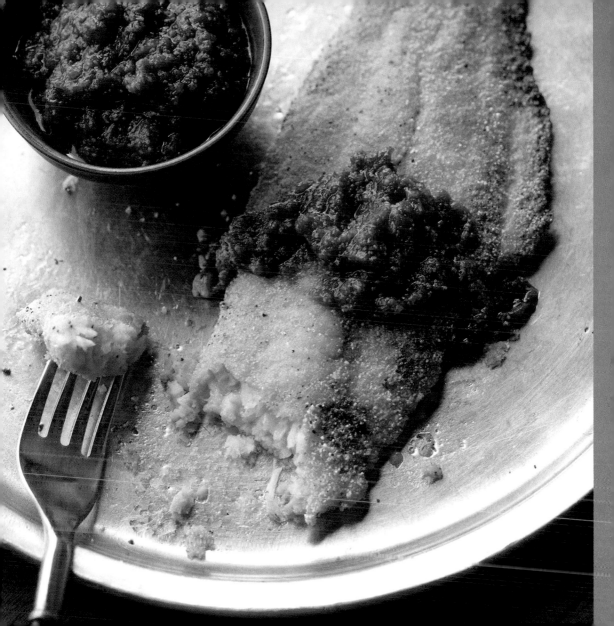

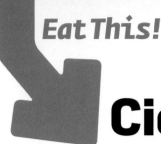

Cioppino

In the late 19th and early 20th centuries, a flood of Italian immigrants made their way to San Francisco, leaving a permanent mark on the culinary fabric of the city. One of the great dishes to come from that period is cioppino, a hearty fish and shellfish soup based on the classic seafood soups of the old country. This is a very fast, very delicious version, combining a full roster of nutritional superstars: tomatoes, garlic, wine, herbs, and lots of fresh seafood.

You'll Need:

- 1 Tbsp olive oil
- 1 bulb fennel, cored and diced, fronds chopped and reserved for garnish
- 1 medium onion, diced
- 4 cloves garlic, roughly chopped
- ½ tsp fennel seeds
- ½ tsp red pepper flakes
- 1 can (28 oz) whole peeled tomatoes
- 1½ cups clam juice
- 1 cup low-sodium chicken broth
- 1½ cups red wine (Pinot)
- 2 bay leaves
- ½ tsp dried thyme
- 1 lb firm white fish, such as halibut, cod, or mahi mahi
- ½ lb medium shrimp, peeled and deveined
- 12 to 16 mussels, scrubbed and debearded
- **Salt and black pepper to taste**

Most mussels come fully cleaned these days, but just in case, pick through and remove any stringy "beards" that may still be attached to the shells.

How to Make It:

- Heat the olive oil in large saucepan or pot over medium heat. Add the fennel, onion, garlic, fennel seeds, and red pepper flakes and sauté for about 5 minutes, until the vegetables are soft.

- Drain the tomatoes, discarding the juice. Lightly crush the tomatoes with your fingers (careful, juice may splatter from inside the tomato). Add the tomatoes to the pot, along with the clam juice, chicken broth, wine, bay leaves, and thyme, and bring to a simmer. Cook for 5 minutes, then add the fish, shrimp, and mussels. Cook for about 5 minutes, until the fish is firm, the shrimp is pink, and the mussels have opened. Discard any mussels that do not open. Taste and adjust seasoning with salt and black pepper.

- Discard the bay leaves and serve the soup with the reserved fennel fronds for garnish.

Makes 6 servings

Per Serving
$4.50
280 calories
6 g fat
(1 g saturated)
760 mg sodium

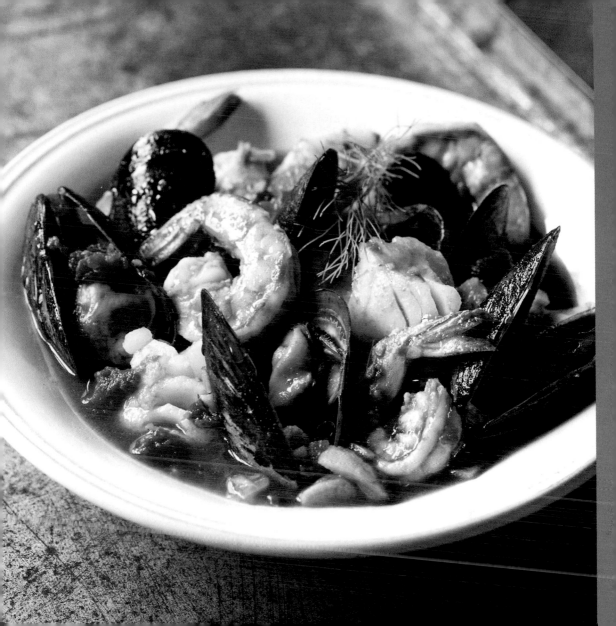

Eat This!

Blackened Tilapia with Garlic-Lime Butter

Ever eaten any blackened food that wasn't delicious (besides those steaks your dad scorches every year at the Fourth of July barbecue)? Neither have we. Consider it a bonus that blackening is actually an incredibly healthy way of cooking, giving the fish or meat a body armor of potent disease-fighting antioxidants in the form of tantalizing spices. Truth be told, the flavored butter here is the icing on the cake; if you have a great fresh piece of fish, just coat it with a bit of blackening spice, follow the cooking instructions, and maybe squeeze a lemon over the top.

You'll Need:

- 2 Tbsp butter, softened at room temperature
- 2 Tbsp chopped fresh cilantro
- 2 cloves garlic, finely minced
- 1 tsp lime zest, plus juice of 1 lime
- 1 Tbsp canola oil
- 4 tilapia fillets (6 oz each)
- 1 Tbsp Magic Blackening Rub (see page 320)

How to Make It:

- Combine the butter, cilantro, garlic, lime zest, and lime juice in a small mixing bowl and stir to thoroughly blend. Set aside.
- Heat the oil in a large cast-iron skillet or sauté pan over high heat. Rub the tilapia all over with the blackening rub. When the oil in the pan lightly smokes, add the fish and cook, undisturbed, for 3 to 4 minutes on the first side, until the spice rub becomes dark and crusty. Flip and continue cooking for 1 to 2 minutes, until the fillets flake with gentle pressure from your finger.
- Transfer the fish to 4 serving plates and immediately top each with a bit of the flavored butter.

Makes 4 servings

Per Serving

$2.32

300 calories
14 g fat
(6 g saturated)
510 mg sodium

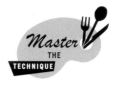

Master THE **TECHNIQUE**

Blackening

The best way to get the full sear you want is in a scorching-hot cast-iron skillet. Heat a thin film of oil in the skillet over the highest possible heat (and turn on the kitchen fan). When wisps of smoke begin to rise from the oil, carefully add the fish or meat. Don't touch it for at least 2 minutes; you want a dark crust to set in over the protein, and fiddling with the food will prevent this from happening. Cook for 75 percent of the time on one side, then flip and finish on the other.

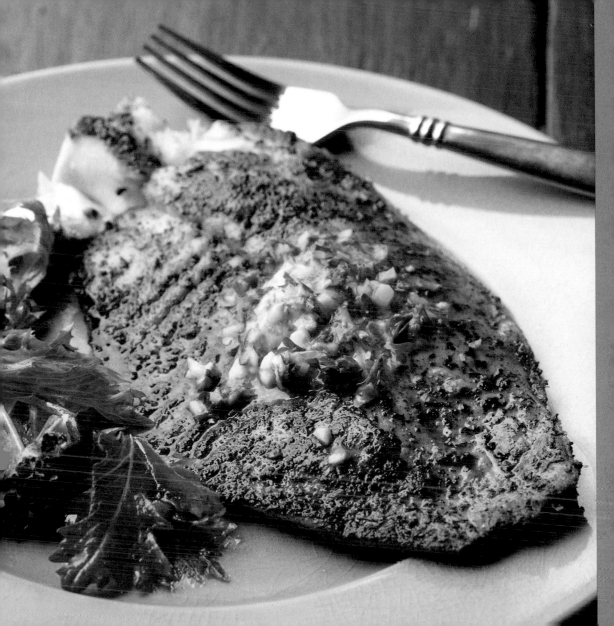

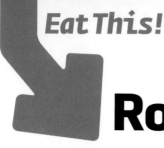

Eat This!

Roast Salmon with Lentils

Lentils have a bit of a PR problem in America. They have been banished to the deepest, darkest parts of the pantry while less-deserving ingredients like rice and pasta get all the love. Truth is, few ingredients fuse nutrition, affordability, ease, and taste quite like the humble lentil. This dish, a bistro classic, is a testament to its greatness. While the salmon roasts away in the oven, the lentils are simmered into tender submission. Separately, each makes for fine eating, but together they merge into something truly special.

You'll Need:

- ½ Tbsp olive oil
- 1 medium carrot, peeled and diced
- ½ medium yellow onion, diced
- 2 cloves garlic, minced
- 1 cup dried lentils
- 3 cups chicken broth or water
- 2 bay leaves
- 2 Tbsp red wine vinegar
- Salt and black pepper to taste
- 4 salmon fillets (4 oz each)
- 2 Tbsp Dijon mustard
- 2 Tbsp brown sugar

How to Make It:

- Preheat the oven to 450°F.
- Heat the olive oil in a medium saucepan over medium heat. Add the carrot, onion, and garlic and sauté for 5 to 7 minutes, until soft and lightly browned. Add the lentils, broth, and bay leaves. Simmer for about 20 minutes, until the lentils are tender and the liquid has mostly evaporated. Before serving, add the vinegar, season with salt and pepper, and discard the bay leaves.
- While the lentils simmer, roast the salmon: Season the fish with salt and black pepper. Combine the mustard and brown sugar in a mixing bowl and spread evenly over the salmon fillets.
- Place the salmon on a baking sheet and place on the top rack of the oven. Roast for 8 to 10 minutes, until the salmon has browned on the surface and flakes with gentle pressure from your finger.
- Divide the lentils among 4 plates or pasta bowls and top each serving with a piece of salmon.

Makes 4 servings

Per Serving
$3.35
440 calories
12 g fat
(2 g saturated)
680 mg sodium

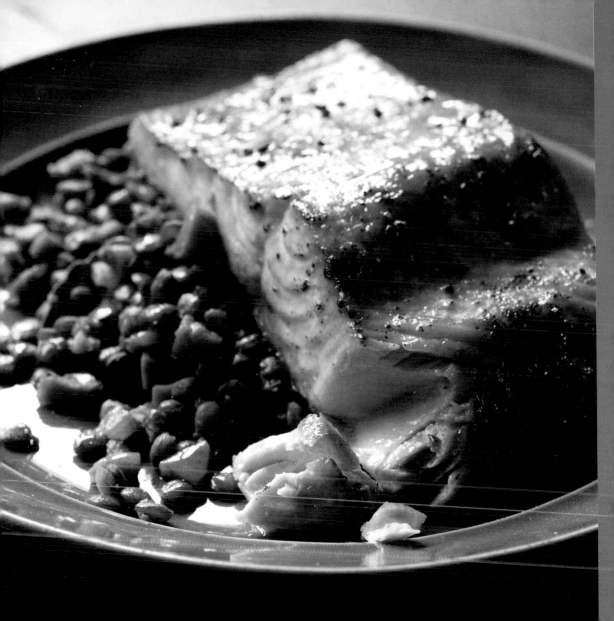

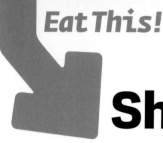

Shrimp & Grits

Most shrimp that shows up on restaurant menus is either breaded and fried or sautéed in a bath of melted butter. Instead, we spike sautéed shrimp with scallions, cayenne, and crispy hunks of kielbasa to keep the calories below 400 in this savory bowl of Southern comfort.

You'll Need:

- 1 Tbsp canola oil
- 1 cup diced cooked turkey kielbasa
- 4 scallions, whites and greens separated, chopped
- 1 clove garlic, minced
- 8 oz fresh mushrooms (button, cremini, or shiitake), stems removed, sliced
- 1 pound shrimp, peeled and deveined
- ½ cup low-sodium chicken broth
- Salt and black pepper to taste
- ½ tsp cayenne pepper
- ½ cup quick-cooking grits
- ¼ cup shredded Cheddar cheese

How to Make It:

- Heat the oil in a large cast-iron skillet or saute pan over medium-high heat until lightly smoking. Add the kielbasa; cook for a few minutes, until lightly browned. Add the scallion whites, garlic, and mushrooms. Cook until the mushrooms are lightly browned, 3 to 4 minutes.
- Add the shrimp and continue cooking until the shrimp are just pink and firm to the touch. Stir in the broth and cook for another 3 minutes, until the liquid has reduced by half and the shrimp are cooked all the way through. Season with salt, pepper, and cayenne.
- While the shrimp are cooking, cook the grits according to the package instructions. When they're thick and creamy, add the cheese and season with salt and pepper.
- Divide the grits and shrimp among 4 bowls and garnish with the scallion greens.

Makes 4 servings

Master THE TECHNIQUE

Deveining shrimp

That vein people always refer to when talking about shrimp? It's actually their digestive tract. You're definitely going to want to cut it out. Here's how.

- **STEP 1:** Peel the shell and remove the tail.
- **STEP 2:** Make a shallow incision along the back.
- **STEP 3:** Fish out the vein with the tip of your knife.

Per Serving

$3.24

340 calories
10 g fat
(4 g saturated)
610 mg sodium

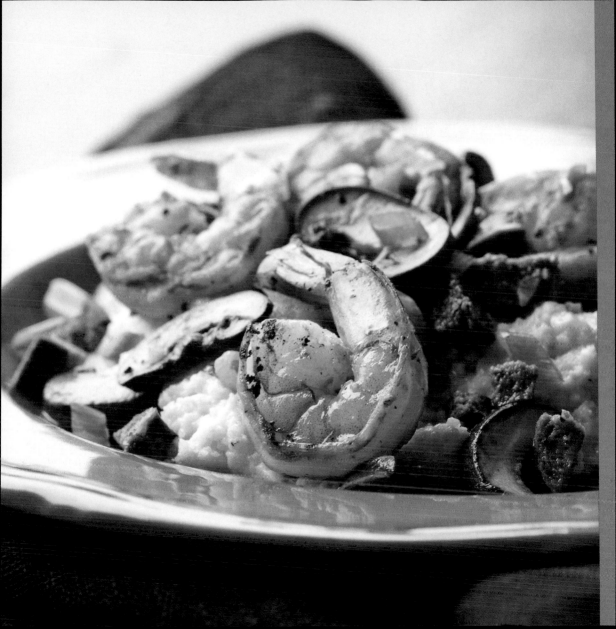

Grilled Swordfish with Caponata

Sicilian cooking is some of the greatest on the planet, built around a tradition of humble pasta dishes, sophisticated desserts, and beautiful fish and seafood preparations. There are two items you will find on nearly every restaurant menu across the island: grilled swordfish and caponata, Sicily's answer to ratatouille, a slow-cooked sweet-and-sour vegetable stew. You rarely see them together in the same dish, but as soon as you taste this—preferably in the summer, with the fish hot off the grill—you'll see why it makes us so happy.

You'll Need:

- 1 Tbsp olive oil, plus more for coating the fish
- 2 medium eggplants, cut into ½" cubes
- 1 medium onion, diced
- 2 cloves garlic, minced
- 1 can (14½ oz) diced tomatoes
- 2 Tbsp raisins (preferably golden raisins)
- 2 Tbsp capers
- 2 Tbsp red wine vinegar
- 1 Tbsp sugar
- ¼ cup chopped fresh basil
- Salt and black pepper to taste
- 4 small swordfish steaks, 6 oz each

How to Make It:

- Heat the olive oil in a medium saucepan over medium heat. Add the eggplant, onion, and garlic and sauté for about 5 minutes, until lightly browned and softened. Add the tomatoes, raisins, capers, vinegar, and sugar. Cover and simmer for 15 minutes, until the vegetables are very soft and the mixture has the consistency of marmalade. Stir in the basil and season with salt and black pepper. Keep warm.

- Preheat a grill or grill pan over medium-high heat. Coat the swordfish with olive oil and season both sides with salt and black pepper. Grill the steaks for 4 minutes, until nice grill marks have developed (you can rotate the steaks 45 degrees midway through to create diamond-shape grill marks if you like). Flip and continue cooking for about 4 minutes longer, until the flesh flakes with gentle pressure from your finger. Serve each serving of swordfish with a generous scoop of caponata over the top.

Makes 4 servings

Per Serving
$5.80
360 calories
11 g fat
(2.5 g saturated)
520 mg sodium

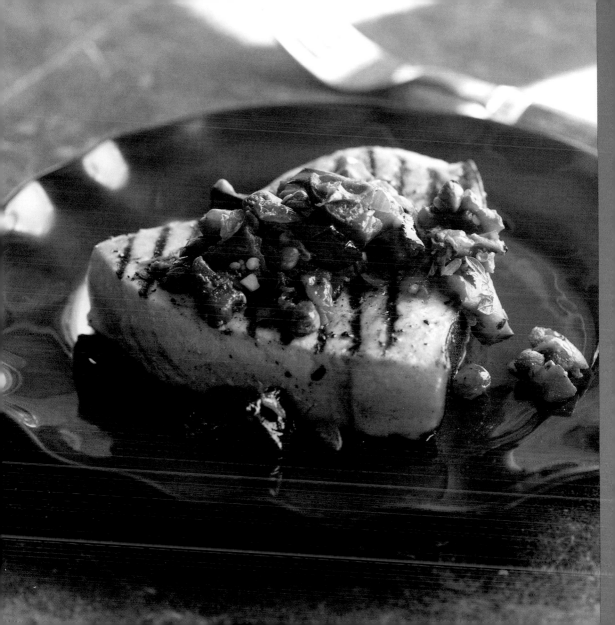

Eat This!

Seared Scallops with White Beans & Spinach

You have to look long and hard to find a scallop on a restaurant menu and we can't quite figure out why. They're a tremendous source of lean protein, super-easy to cook, and stack up well with bold and subtle flavors alike. Learn to properly sear a scallop (hint: make sure the scallop is very dry and the pan is very hot) and you'll be won over.

You'll Need:

- 2 strips bacon, chopped into small pieces
- ½ red onion, minced
- 1 clove garlic, minced
- 1 can (14 oz) white beans, rinsed and drained
- 4 cups baby spinach
- 1 lb large sea scallops

Salt and black pepper to taste

- 1 Tbsp butter

Juice of 1 lemon

Feel free to kill the bacon, but for about 18 calories per serving, it adds a ton of flavor to the overall dish.

There are a lot of different types of white beans sold in cans. All will work, but cannellini beans are best.

How to Make It:

- Heat a medium saucepan over low heat. Cook the bacon until it has begun to crisp. Add the onion and garlic; saute until the onion is soft and translucent, 2 to 3 minutes. Add the beans and spinach and simmer until the beans are hot and the spinach is wilted. Keep warm.

- Heat a large cast-iron skillet or saute pan over medium-high heat. Blot the scallops dry with a paper towel and season with salt and pepper on both sides. Add the butter and the scallops to the pan and sear the scallops for 2 to 3 minutes per side, until deeply caramelized.

- Before serving, add the lemon juice to the beans. Season with salt and pepper. Divide the beans among 4 warm bowls or plates and top with scallops.

Makes 4 servings

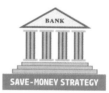

SAVE-MONEY STRATEGY

Sea scallops in the seafood case can be pricey, but scallops—like shrimp—rarely arrive at the market fresh. Instead, they're frozen after catching and defrosted when put on sale. So why pay the extra cash for faux-fresh scallops when you can buy them frozen for a fraction of the price? Grocers like Trader Joe's and Whole Foods sell bags of high-quality frozen scallops and shrimp for about 60 percent of the seafood-case cost.

Per Serving
$4.15
280 calories
7 g fat
(2.5 g saturated)
360 mg sodium

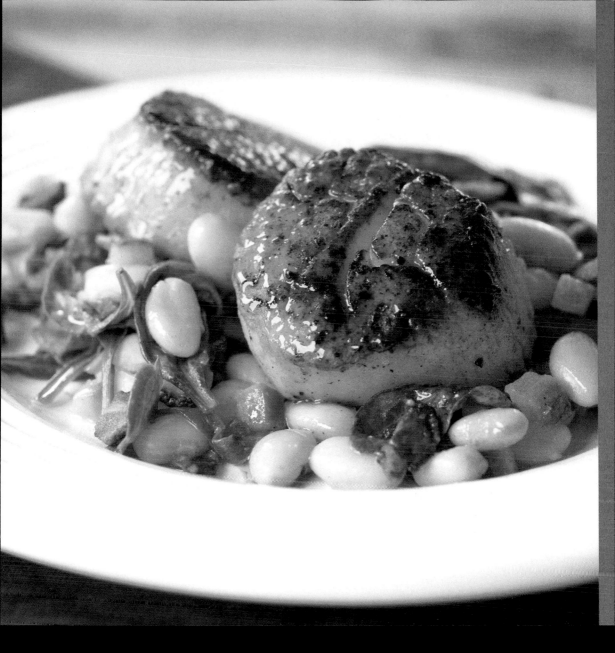

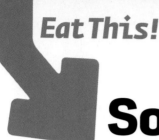

Sole Meunière

Deadly simple but intensely satisfying, this French bistro classic ranks as one of the great dishes of the world—especially when made with the freshest fish possible. Sole is extremely tough to come by in most parts of America, and it's known to inflict damage to the wallet, so we recommend trying this with flounder, which is widely available at about half the price. The French might not approve, but it will be our little secret.

You'll Need:

- 4 fillets sole or flounder (6 oz each)
- Salt to taste
- ¼ cup flour
- 4 Tbsp butter
- Juice and zest of 1 lemon
- Chopped fresh parsley

How to Make It:

- Season the fish on both sides with salt. Place the flour in a flat dish and dredge the fish on both sides, shaking off any excess flour.
- Heat 2 tablespoons of the butter in a large nonstick pan over medium heat until foaming and lightly browned (careful, butter goes from brown to burnt very quickly). Working in two batches if necessary, cook the fish, turning once, for about 6 minutes total, until it's nicely browned on both sides and flakes with gentle pressure from your finger. Place a fillet on each of 4 warm plates.
- Add the remaining 2 tablespoons butter, the lemon juice and zest, and parsley to the pan. Swirl the pan until the butter is fully melted. Divide the sauce among the 4 fillets and serve.

Makes 4 servings

Per Serving
$3.91
290 calories
14 g fat
(8 g saturated)
460 mg sodium

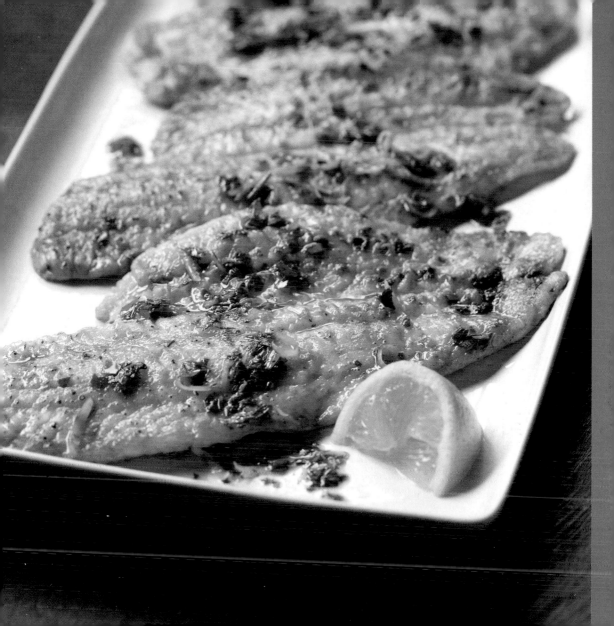

CHAPTER 10

INTERNATIONAL

America's Worst ETHNIC FOODS

**PF Chang's
Kung Pao Chicken**

960 calories
58 g fat
(9 g saturated)
1,430 mg sodium
Price: $13.95

"Kung pao" sounds like a fierce martial arts move, which is appropriate considering it might chop your chances of sporting a flat belly. The bird is battered and fried—the one-two punch responsible for the undoing of most Asian-style chicken dishes. Chinese food is usually associated with takeout, but if you take it in—to your home kitchen, that is—you can create a much less oily opponent.

Eat This Instead!
Kung Pao Chicken
(page 288)

290 calories
13 g fat (2 g saturated)
670 mg sodium
Cost per serving: $1.96

Save! 670 calories and $11.99!

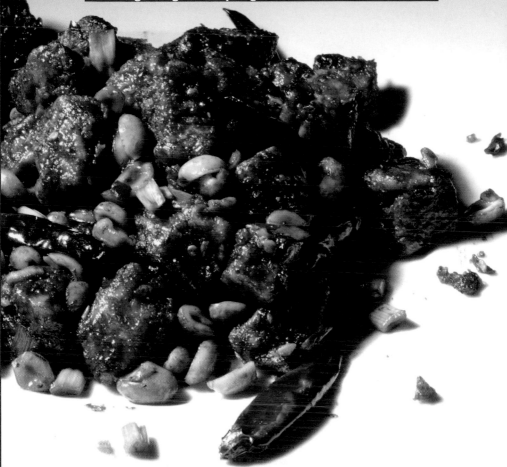

960 calories

PF Chang's Kung Pao hits your gut like a Chuck Norris roundhouse.

Panda Express's Beijing Beef (with fried rice)

990 calories
42 g fat
(8 g saturated)
1,510 mg sodium
Price: $5.49

It's not often that red meat gets a piping-hot oil bath, which—if this Panda Express dish is any indication—is good news for your waistline. The battered beef here is the worst Panda has to offer, and its sweet sauce—a frequent offender on Asian-American menus—contributes more than a Twix Bar's worth of sugar. Nearly as bad as the beef is the rice, which adds a staggering 530 calories to this dish on its own, a reminder that starch—as much as oil and salt—is a killer at Chinese restaurants.

Eat This Instead!
Beef with Broccoli
(page 282)

330 calories
13 g fat (4 g saturated)
900 mg sodium
Cost per serving: $3.23
Save! 660 calories and $2.26!

WORST STEAK
Cheesecake Factory's Steak Diane with Fries

2,010 calories
N/A g fat (47 g saturated fat)
3,018 mg sodium
Price: $19.95

According to our research, Steak Diane is named after Diana, Roman goddess of the heft—err—hunt. But regardless of its namesake, the French-American specialty is fried in butter and swimming in cream, so it comes as no surprise that the Factory's version breaks the 2,000-calorie mark. Swap this meal for our French-style steak and french fries just once a week and you could save 24 pounds and $851 in a year.

Eat This Instead!
Steak Frites with Compound Butter (page 276)

460 calories
24 g fat (11 g saturated)
660 mg sodium
Cost per serving: $3.57
Save! 1,550 calories and $16.38!

WORST MEXICAN
On the Border's Ranchiladas (with refried beans)

1,260 calories
66 g fat (34 g saturated)
3,180 mg sodium
Price: $9.99

Enchiladas have always been a humble home-cooked comfort staple across Mexico, but when they resurface on Tex-Mex menus in America, the reality gets a bit murkier. On the Border takes what should be a beautifully simple dish—shredded chicken wrapped in a corn tortilla and covered in salsa—and muddies up the concept with excess cheese, creamy sauce, massive portions, and sorry sides. Grab a rotisserie chicken, a package of corn tortillas, and a bottle of salsa and return the enchilada to its rightful place as a lean and satisfying comfort food.

Eat This Instead!
Chicken and Red Chile Enchiladas (page 270)

375 calories
12 g fat (5 g saturated)
630 mg sodium
Cost per serving: $1.83
Save! 885 calories and $8.16!

WORST CHINESE BEEF ENTRÉE
PF Chang's Long Life Noodles with Prawns

1,040 calories
37 g fat (11 g saturated)
3,830 mg sodium
Price: $11.25

With a name like this, it's hard not to expect a bit of trouble. But a plate of noodles with more sodium than 14 large orders of McDonald's french fries crosses the threshold from disappointing to down-right dangerous. At its best, Chinese cuisine is one of the healthiest on the planet, but these noodles illustrate the many perils of eating it outside of your own home.

Eat This Instead!
Sesame Noodles with Chicken (page 284)

340 calories
11 g fat (2 g saturated)
400 mg sodium
Cost per serving: $2.05
Save! 700 calories and $9.20!

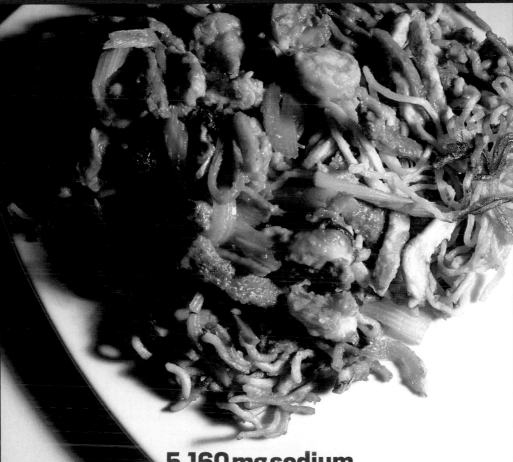

5,160 mg sodium

PF Chang's Double Pan-Fried Noodles: enough calories to feed a family and enough salt to preserve a whole hog!

Mortar & Pestle

Admit it: At some point you've caved to the dubious promise of some whiz-bang new piece of kitchen gadgetry. Maybe it was late at night and you ordered a bread knife capable of sawing through a Master Lock. Or perhaps some smarmy pitchman at the mall convinced you to buy a 12-gallon margarita machine that now gathers dust in your attic. Forgive yourself. Your intentions were good. But realize this: While the Ron Popeils and Cutcos of the world try to reinvent the wheel, one tool has proven impervious to technological advancement or entrepreneurial tinkering: the mortar and pestle.

The simplicity is almost off-putting. It's essentially a bowl and a stick. But there's a reason why it continues to be one of the most important tools in kitchens from Thailand to Spain to Mexico: Together, the bowl and stick are vital for unlocking layers of flavor, whether mashing garlic into smooth purées, smashing herbs into aromatic pastes, or pulverizing dried spices into potent powders.

So why not use a spice grinder or a food processor? Three reasons: The fast-moving blades can bruise soft leaves, the heat-generating motor can burn off delicate oils, and the machines are intrinsically more difficult to clean. The mortar and pestle move only as fast as your hand, generate a negligible amount of friction heat, and require cleaning that is as simple as wiping down with a clean rag.

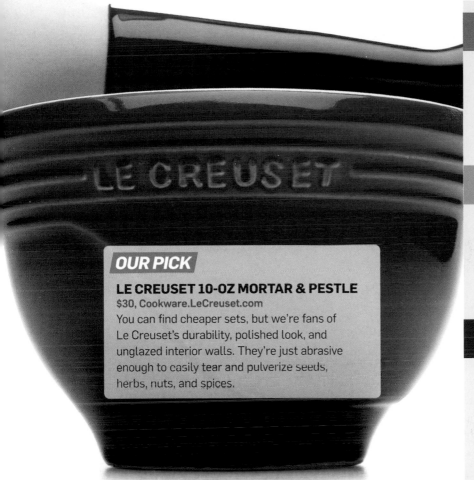

Mortar &Pestle *SUPERPOWERS*

LEARN TO SALSA

The best salsa and guacamole come from a mortar and pestle. Start by mashing garlic with a pinch of salt, then add in cilantro and onion, then either chopped tomatoes (for salsa) or fresh avocado (for guac). Finish with a squeeze of lime and serve directly from the mortar.

WAKE UP YOUR SPICES

Whole spices have more flavor than the pre-ground stuff you find in bottles. Buy whole seeds like coriander, cumin, and cardamom and crush them up just before cooking. Dried chiles and whole peppercorns will add more punch after they've been bashed up in a mortar.

DOUBLE THE FLAVOR OF FRESH HERBS

Muddle mint for mojitos, crush basil (along with garlic, pine nuts, and olive oil) into pesto, or bash up cilantro, parsley, or oregano just before garnishing pasta or soup.

OUR PICK

LE CREUSET 10-OZ MORTAR & PESTLE
$30, Cookware.LeCreuset.com

You can find cheaper sets, but we're fans of Le Creuset's durability, polished look, and unglazed interior walls. They're just abrasive enough to easily tear and pulverize seeds, herbs, nuts, and spices.

The Wok Matrix

Wok cooking goes back nearly as far as cavemen roasting meat on sticks, and even after thousands of years of culinary advancements, it remains one of the quickest, most efficient, unfussiest, and delicious cooking forms on the planet. Once you learn a few basic principles and map out your favorite flavor profiles, you can wok your way to hundreds of different meals—all with little to no forethought and only a few minutes of concentrated cooking.

Four Master Stir-Fries

It's nearly impossible to make a bad stir-fry with the ingredients laid out to the right. These combinations just happen to be some of our favorites.

CHOOSE YOUR PROTEIN

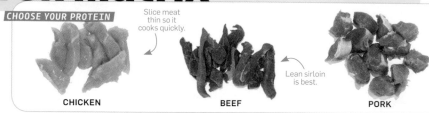

Slice meat thin so it cooks quickly.

Lean sirloin is best.

CHICKEN **BEEF** **PORK**

CHOOSE YOUR VEGETABLES

SLICED ONION **CHOPPED EGGPLANT** **CHOPPED BROCCOLI** **SLICED BELL PEPPERS**

CHOOSE YOUR SAUCE

Figure 1 tablespoon of any sauce per serving.

CHILI GARLIC **BLACK BEAN** **SWEET & SOUR**

CHOOSE YOUR GARNISH

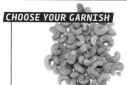 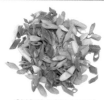

ROASTED CASHEWS **CHOPPED PEANUTS** **SLICED SCALLIONS**

CHILI GARLIC PORK
Pork + onion + bell pepper + chili garlic sauce + scallions

BLACK BEAN CHICKEN
Chicken + zucchini + eggplant + black bean sauce + cilantro

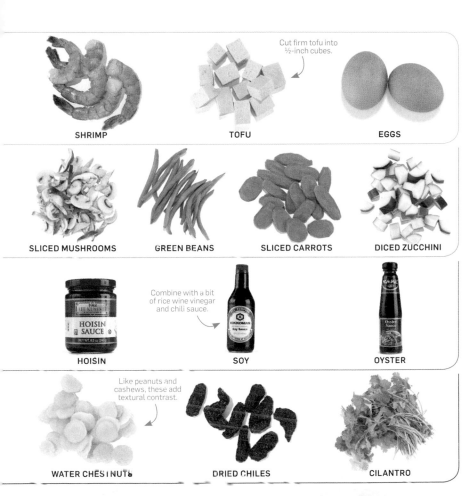

Cut firm tofu into ½-inch cubes.

SHRIMP

TOFU

EGGS

SLICED MUSHROOMS

GREEN BEANS

SLICED CARROTS

DICED ZUCCHINI

Combine with a bit of rice wine vinegar and chili sauce.

HOISIN

SOY

OYSTER

Like peanuts and cashews, these add textural contrast.

WATER CHESTNUTS

DRIED CHILES

CILANTRO

BROCCOLI BEEF
Beef + broccoli + bell pepper
+ oyster sauce + water chestnuts

VEGETARIAN FEAST
Tofu + eggplant + zucchini + carrots
+ broccoli + hoisin

The Rules of the Wok

Crank the heat
Add just enough oil (peanut or canola) to coat the wok—1 to 2 tablespoons. When the oil is hot, add the protein and cook it until it changes color, moving it constantly with a wooden spoon or metal spatula to ensure even cooking. Remove the protein and set it aside.

Build a base
Use a paper towel and tongs to wipe out the wok. Add a touch more oil and when hot, add a teaspoon each of thinly sliced ginger and garlic and cook until fragrant—15 seconds or so.

Cook hard and fast
Add your vegetables and cook them for 3 to 4 minutes. Again, it's important to keep things moving with your spoon or spatula. A perfectly stir-fried vegetable is fork tender with a little crunch.

Set your sauce
Return the protein to the wok. Most Chinese chefs add a ⅓ cup of broth and a pinch of cornstarch. Cook over high heat until the broth thickens, about 1 minute, then stir in your sauce. Cook for another minute, garnish, and eat.

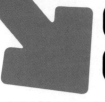

Chicken & Red Chile Enchiladas

We'd love to bag on restaurant-style enchiladas, but truth is, even in the worst Mexican chain restaurants, enchiladas are normally your safest bet—as long they're made with corn tortillas (lighter than flour), filled with shredded chicken (better than ground beef), and covered in salsa and a layer of cheese (gentler than the battery of condiments that cover most Mexican dishes). Play with the filling as you see fit, but this is the blueprint for enchilada success.

You'll Need:

- 1 can (28 oz) whole peeled tomatoes, excess liquid poured off
- 1 onion, peeled and thinly sliced
- 2 cloves garlic
- 2 Tbsp chipotle pepper
- 1 tsp cumin

Pinch of cinnamon (optional)

Salt and black pepper to taste

- ½ Tbsp canola or peanut oil
- 2 cups shredded chicken, preferably from a store-bought rotisserie chicken
- 12 corn tortillas
- 1 cup shredded Jack cheese

Fresh cilantro for garnish (optional)

How to Make It:

- Combine the tomatoes, half the onion, the garlic, chipotle, cumin, and cinnamon (if using) in a blender. Puree until smooth. Season with salt and black pepper. Preheat the oven to 375°F.

- Heat the oil in a saucepan over medium heat. Add the sauce and simmer for 15 minutes. Spread one-third of the sauce on the bottom of a 13" x 9" baking dish. Combine the chicken with another third of the sauce in a mixing bowl.

- Wrap the tortillas in a damp kitchen towel and microwave for 30 seconds, until hot and pliable. Arrange a few generous tablespoons of sauced chicken down the center of a tortilla and gently roll up. Place the filled tortilla seam-side down in the baking dish. Repeat with the remaining chicken and tortillas.

- Cover the enchiladas with the remaining sauce and top with the cheese. Bake for 10 to 12 minutes, until the cheese is melted. Top the enchiladas with the remaining onion slices and cilantro, if you like, before serving.

Makes 6 servings

Per Serving

$1.83

375 calories
12 g fat
(5 g saturated)
630 mg sodium

MEAL MULTIPLIER

Other ways to construct an enchilada masterpiece:

- Fill with grilled zucchini, peppers, and onions and top with bottled salsa verde and Jack cheese.

- Fill with grilled shrimp and black beans and top with bottled salsa verde.

- Fill with Braised Brisket (page 230) and follow the instructions in this recipe.

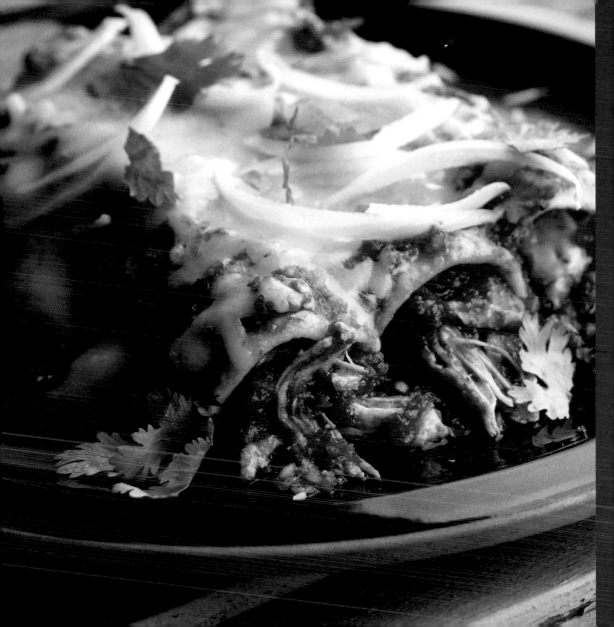

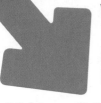

Vegetable Fried Rice with a Fried Egg

Making a dish like fried rice healthy requires the same strategy employed when lightening a bowl of pasta: The add-ins need to be more abundant than the carbs themselves. Use any mixture of firm vegetables you have in your refrigerator (the more the merrier!), just be sure to cut them into similar-size pieces so they cook in the same amount of time. Eggs are normally scrambled directly into the rice, where they get lost in the jumble of grains and soy. We prefer a single, just-cooked egg on top; break the yolk and dig in.

You'll Need:

- 1 Tbsp canola or peanut oil
- 2 cloves garlic, minced
- 1 Tbsp minced fresh ginger
- 4 cups chopped vegetables, such as asparagus, broccoli, carrot, bell pepper, zucchini, snap peas, green beans, onions (the more variety the better)
- 4 cups cooked brown rice, cooled
- 2 Tbsp low-sodium soy sauce
- 4 eggs, fried sunny side up

Sriracha for serving

How to Make It:

- Heat the oil in a large wok or nonstick skillet over high heat. When the oil is lightly smoking, add the garlic, ginger, and chopped vegetables. Stir-fry the vegetables for about 5 minutes, until lightly browned and softened, using a spatula to keep the ingredients moving so that they cook evenly.

- Add the rice and cook, stirring, for another 3 minutes, then add the soy sauce and cook for 1 minute more. (If you like crispy bits in your fried rice, leave the rice to cook, undisturbed, for 1 minute. A nice crust should form on the bottom layer of rice.)

- Divide the fried rice among 4 plates or bowls and top each with a fried egg. Serve with sriracha.

Makes 4 servings

Per Serving
$1.31
360 calories
12 g fat
(2.5 g saturated)
390 mg sodium

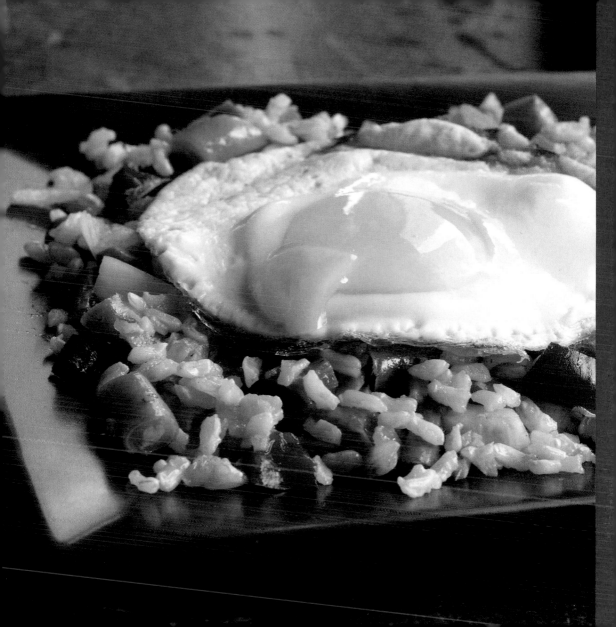

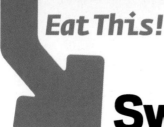

Swedish Meatballs

We're used to our meatballs coming in a vat of bubbling red sauce, but that's a very narrow definition of a food so diversely interpreted throughout the world. Swedes have been forming spheres of beef and veal and covering them in sauce for hundreds of years, and when Scandinavian immigrants landed in the Midwest, they brought this taste of home with them. This version cuts the beef with turkey, which is tender and light like veal, but considerably leaner.

You'll Need:

2   slices white bread, torn into tiny pieces

½   cup 2% milk

12 oz ground chuck

12 oz ground turkey

1   small onion, minced

2   cloves garlic, minced

½   tsp ground nutmeg

1   tsp salt

¼   tsp black pepper

1   Tbsp butter

2   Tbsp flour

1½ cups low-sodium beef stock

1   Tbsp Greek yogurt

Cranberry or raspberry marmalade for serving (optional)

How to Make It:

● Combine the bread and ¼ cup of the milk in a bowl and soak for 5 minutes. Drain and use your hands to squeeze out some of the liquid absorbed by the bread (you want it to be moist, not sopping). In a mixing bowl, combine the bread with the beef, turkey, onion, garlic, nutmeg, salt, and pepper. Gently mix, then form into golf ball-sized meatballs.

● Heat the butter in a large nonstick sauté pan or skillet over medium heat. Add the meatballs and cook, turning occasionally, for about 10 minutes, until nicely browned on all sides and cooked through. Remove the meatballs to a plate and reserve.

● Add the flour to the pan, stirring with a whisk or a wooden spoon to incorporate evenly into the remaining fat. Add the stock slowly, stirring frequently to keep lumps from forming. Add the remaining ¼ cup milk and simmer for about 3 minutes, until the flour begins to thicken the liquid. Stir in the yogurt, then return the meatballs to the pan, cooking for about 10 minutes longer, until the sauce clings tightly to the meatballs. Serve by themselves, or with boiled potatoes or lightly buttered noodles. Pass the marmalade at the table, if using.

Makes 6 servings

Per Serving
$1.45
280 calories
15 g fat
(6 g saturated)
700 mg sodium

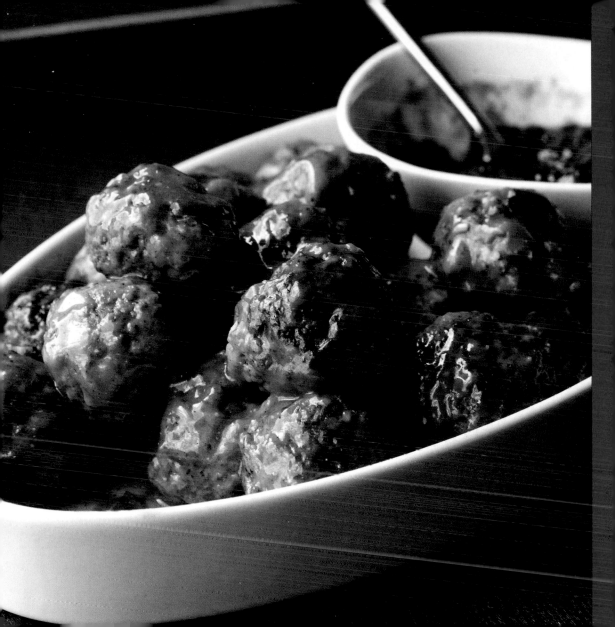

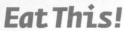

Steak Frites with Compound Butter

At Le Relais de Venise in Paris, people line up around the block for a taste of some of the city's best steak frites. Inside, it's all business: A crew of stone-faced female servers in French maid outfits serve up nothing but beef (entrecôte, cooked to the rosy side of red) and potatoes (thin and crispy), all covered in an herb-spiked butter sauce that will haunt you for months to come. This is our nod to meat and potatoes done the French way.

You'll Need:

- 4 Tbsp butter, softened
- Juice of ½ lemon
- 1 small shallot, minced
- 1 clove garlic, peeled and grated
- 1 Tbsp minced fresh chives
- 1 tsp Dijon mustard
- 1 tsp Worcestershire
- 1 lb skirt or hanger steak
- Salt and black pepper to taste
- Crispy Oven-Baked Fries (page 298)

How to Make It:

- Combine the butter, lemon juice, shallot, garlic, chives, mustard, and Worcestershire in a mixing bowl. Stir to thoroughly combine. Reserve on the countertop.
- Preheat a grill, grill pan, or cast-iron skillet over high heat. Season the steak all over with salt and plenty of black pepper. Cook the steaks, turning frequently, for about 8 minutes total (depending on the thickness), until well browned on both sides and firm but still easily yielding to the touch. Rest for at least 5 minutes before slicing. Top each steak with one-fourth of the butter and serve with the hot fries.

Makes 4 servings

You can use any cut of steak you like here, but the texture and beefiness of skirt or hanger steak most closely captures the cuts of steak commonly used in the classic French brasseries of Paris.

Punch up the butter an extra notch by adding 2 tablespoons of crumbled blue cheese. Form it into a log using plastic wrap and store in the refrigerator for up to 2 weeks.

Per Serving
$3.57
460 calories
24 g fat
(11 g saturated)
660 mg sodium

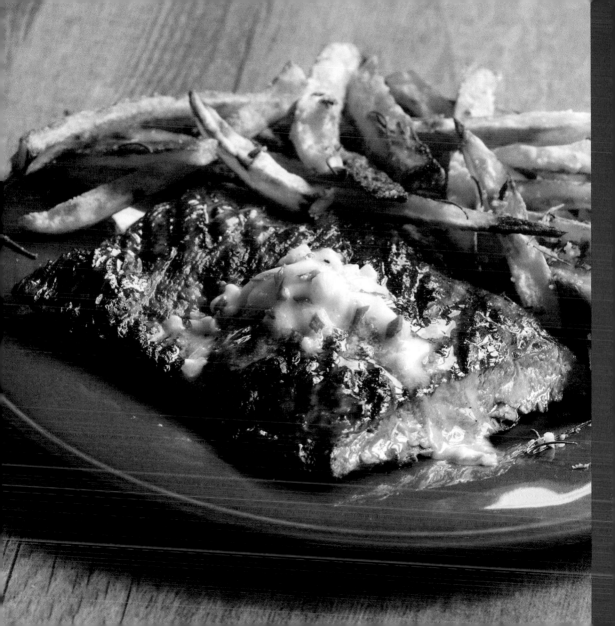

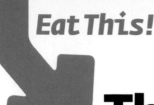

Thai Chicken Curry

Redolent of ginger and lemongrass, chiles and coconut milk, Thai curry brings all of the classic flavors of Southeast Asian cuisine—salty, sour, bitter, hot—together in one dish. What's more, it derives all of its flavor from ingredients packed with powerful antioxidants. Even coconut milk contains lauric acid, among the healthiest forms of fat you can consume. The flavors may be exotic, but the tender chicken, the bouquet of vegetables, and the rich coconut milk will all taste wonderfully familiar.

You'll Need:

- 1 Tbsp peanut or canola oil
- 1 large onion, sliced
- 2 cloves garlic, minced
- 2 tsp minced fresh ginger
- 1 Tbsp red curry paste
- 1 can (14 oz) light coconut milk
- 1 cup chicken stock
- 1 large sweet potato, peeled and cut into cubes
- 8 oz green beans
- 1 lb boneless, skinless chicken breasts, sliced into ¼"-thick pieces

Juice of 1 lime

- 1 Tbsp fish sauce (optional)

Chopped fresh cilantro or basil, for garnish

How to Make It:

- Heat the oil in a large saucepan or pot over medium heat. Add the onions, garlic, and ginger and sauté for about 5 minutes, until soft and fragrant. Add the curry paste, cook for a few minutes, then stir in the coconut milk and broth and bring to a simmer.

- Add the sweet potato and simmer for 10 minutes. Stir in the green beans and chicken and cook for about 5 minutes, until the vegetables are just tender and the chicken is cooked through. Stir in the lime juice and fish sauce, if using. Serve over steamed brown rice, garnished with cilantro or basil, if you like.

Makes 4 servings

Per Serving
$3.17
340 calories
13 g fat
(6 g saturated)
400 mg sodium

SECRET WEAPON

Red Curry Paste

Available in Asian markets and the international sections of large grocers, red curry paste is a potent blend of chiles, herbs, and spices that can be used to ratchet up both the flavor and the nutritional profile of common dishes. Try it rubbed on pork or chicken as a pre-grill marinade, stirred into Greek yogurt and lime juice as a dipping sauce for fish, or blended with peanut butter, lime, and coconut milk to make a satay sauce, the Asian-style barbecue sauce of unrivaled depth and complexity.

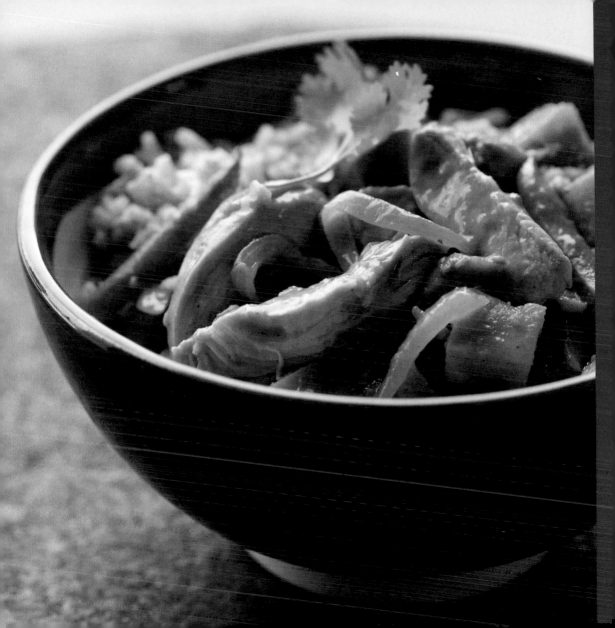

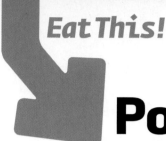

Eat This!

Pork Chile Verde

This isn't a dish that's on most Americans' radar, but it should be—tender pieces of pork stewed in a lively, slightly spicy broth studded with vegetables. Add a few warm tortillas, a hunk of lime, and a cerveza and you're halfway to Mexico with a huge grin on your face. Just make sure you enjoy this one in the comfort and safety of your own kitchen, okay?

You'll Need:

- 1 Tbsp canola oil
- 2 lb boneless pork shoulder, cut into 1" cubes

Salt and black pepper to taste

- 1 cup low-sodium chicken stock
- 1 bottle (15 oz) salsa verde
- 1 medium onion, quartered
- 1 large green bell pepper, chopped into big chunks
- 2 cups small marble or fingerling potatoes (optional)
- 8 corn tortillas
- 2 limes, cut into quarters

Salsa verde is a mild salsa made from onion and tangy tomatillos. Perfect for tacos and eggs.

How to Make It:

- Heat the oil in a large skillet or sauté pan over high heat. Season the pork with salt and pepper. Working in batches, add the pork to the skillet and sear on all sides until caramelized on the outside but still raw in the center (don't over-crowd the pork or it will steam, not brown). Transfer to a slow cooker.

- Add the broth to the hot skillet and use a wooden spoon to scrape up any crispy, flavorful bits of pork. Pour the broth over the pork, along with the salsa verde, onion, and bell pepper. Set the slow cooker to high and cook for 4 hours (or low and cook for 8), until the pork is extremely tender. If using the potatoes, add them to the pot in the final hour of cooking.

- Serve the pork in bowls with the stewed vegetables, along with a ladle of the cooking liquid. Have hot corn tortillas and lime hunks on hand for makeshift tacos.

Makes 6 servings

LEFTOVER♥LOVE

Extra chile verde is an infinite source of inspiration and deliciousness. Start at breakfast: Warm up a small bowl of the leftovers and top with two gently poached eggs. For lunch, serve a scoop over a bowl of black beans and fresh avocado. For dinner, chop the meat and the vegetables and stuff into warm corn tortillas. Top with the stewy liquid and cheese and bake in a 400°F oven for 15 minutes. Finish with slices of raw onion and you have first-class enchiladas.

Per Serving
$2.90
460 calories
24 g fat
(8 g saturated)
620 mg sodium

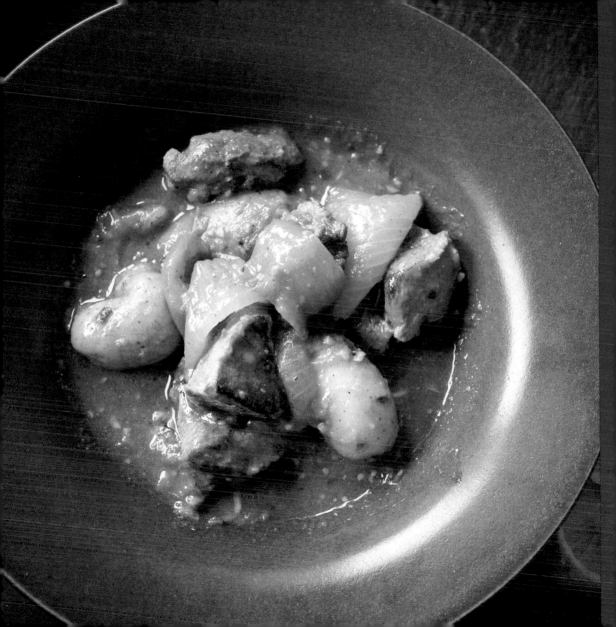

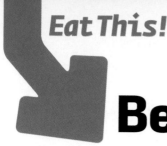

Beef with Broccoli

Beef with broccoli is one of the most recognizable stars in the Chinese-American food galaxy. No doubt it has spent some time hanging out in your refrigerator in a cardboard delivery box—a pile of beef with a few flecks of broccoli buried under a viscous tide of salty brown sauce. This recipe captures the soul of the original recipe, but without all of the excess sauce, oil, and sodium. Instead, count on plenty of lean meat, tons of fresh broccoli, and a delicious sauce that lightly coats the stir-fry.

You'll Need:

- 3 Tbsp low-sodium soy sauce
- 3 Tbsp oyster sauce
- 2 Tbsp Shaoxing rice wine, sherry, or dry white wine
- 1 Tbsp brown sugar
- 1 tsp toasted sesame oil
- 1 tsp cornstarch
- 1 lb flank steak, thinly sliced
- ½ Tbsp canola or peanut oil
- 1 lb broccoli, broken into bite-size pieces
- 1 red or yellow bell pepper, cored and sliced
- 4 cloves garlic, minced
- 1 Tbsp grated fresh ginger
- ¼ cup low-sodium beef stock

How to Make It:

- Combine the soy sauce, oyster sauce, Shaoxing, brown sugar, sesame oil, and cornstarch in a large mixing bowl. Whisk to combine the liquid with the cornstarch. Mix in the beef and let marinate for 30 minutes.
- Heat the oil in a wok over medium heat. Add the broccoli, bell pepper, garlic, and ginger and stir-fry, using a spatula to keep the vegetables moving, for about 5 minutes, until the vegetables have softened. Add the beef and its marinade and continue cooking, stirring frequently, for about 5 minutes, until the beef is browned and nearly cooked through. Add the stock and cook for another 2 minutes, until the sauce thickens and clings to the beef and vegetables. Serve over steamed brown rice, if you like.

Makes 4 servings

Per Serving

$3.23

330 calories

13 g fat
(4 g saturated)

900 mg sodium

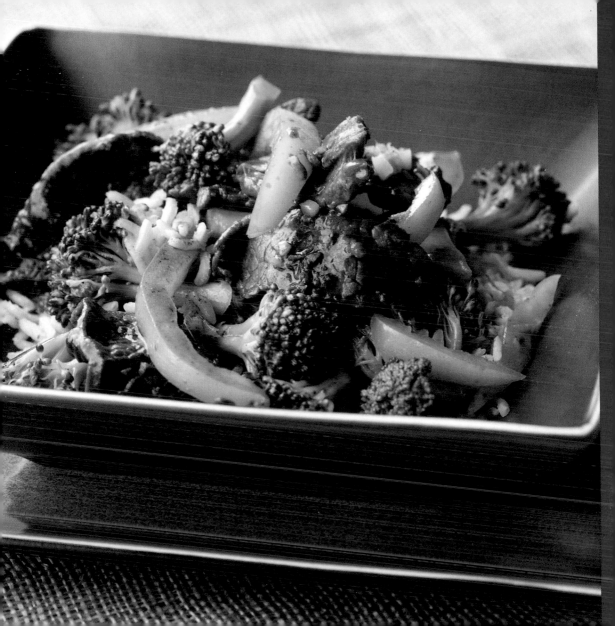

Eat This!

Sesame Noodles with Chicken

Italians might cringe in horror to hear it, but the noodle originally comes from Asia. In 2005, archaeologists discovered what they believe to be the oldest bowl of noodles on record, dating back some 4,000 years. (No word yet on what type of sauce they were dressed with.) The point being that sometimes a box of fettuccine is just as appropriate for an Asian-inspired meal as it is for an Italian repast. Think of this as a salad, with the noodles sitting in for lettuce. Add some protein and as many or as few vegetables as you like, and toss the whole package with a light but powerful dressing. It's the culmination of four millennia of noodle knowledge. (Well, maybe not, but it's awfully tasty.)

You'll Need:

- 6 oz whole-wheat fettuccine
- 2 tsp toasted sesame oil, plus more for noodles

Juice of 1 lime

- 2 Tbsp warm water
- 1½ Tbsp chunky peanut butter
- 1½ Tbsp low-sodium soy sauce
- 2 tsp chili sauce, such as sriracha
- 2 cups shredded chicken

- 1 red or yellow bell pepper, sliced
- 2 cups sugar snap peas
- 1 cup cooked and shelled edamame (optional)

Chopped peanuts, sesame seeds, or chopped scallions (optional)

The sugar snaps work perfectly fine raw in this dish, but if you prefer them cooked, toss them in with the pasta 2 minutes before it finishes cooking. You can do the same with green beans if you can't find sugar snaps.

How to Make It:

- Bring a large pot of salted water to a boil and cook the pasta according to package instructions. Drain the pasta and toss in a large bowl with a bit of sesame oil and rice wine vinegar to keep the noodles from sticking.

- Combine the lime juice, water, peanut butter, soy sauce, chili sauce, and sesame oil in a microwave-safe mixing bowl. Microwave for 45 seconds, then stir to create a uniform sauce.

- Add the sauce to the noodles and toss to mix. Stir in the chicken, bell pepper, sugar snaps, and edamame, if using. Top individual servings with peanuts, sesame seeds, or scallions if you like.

Makes 4 servings

Per Serving

$2.05

340 calories
11 g fat
(2 g saturated)
400 mg sodium

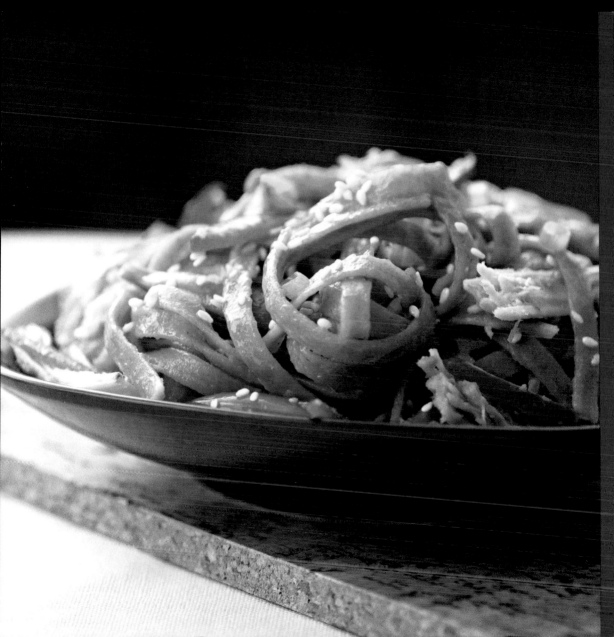

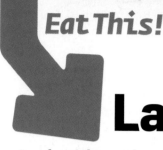

Lamb Tagine

Lamb might not be most Americans' first idea of comfort food, but consider the luxe treatment of this underappreciated protein: lavishly seasoned with the best of the Moroccan spice cabinet, bolstered with golden raisins and fresh ginger, and braised in a slow cooker with a flavorful broth until falling apart. Serve it all up over a soft bed of golden couscous with a ladle of the braising liquid and you begin to understand why lamb is one of the world's most popular meats.

You'll Need:

- 1 Tbsp olive oil
- 2 lb lamb stewing meat (from shoulder or leg)
- Salt and black pepper to taste
- 2 cups low-sodium chicken stock
- 2 large onions, quartered
- 4 carrots, peeled and chopped into ¾" pieces
- 3 Roma tomatoes, seeded and chopped
- 1 Tbsp minced fresh ginger
- 6 cloves garlic, peeled
- 1 tsp cumin
- 1 stick cinnamon (or ½ tsp ground cinnamon)
- ¼ tsp cayenne
- 1 can (15 oz) chickpeas
- ¼ cup golden raisins
- 2 cups cooked couscous
- Chopped cilantro

How to Make It:

- Heat the oil in a large skillet over medium-high heat. Season the lamb all over with salt and pepper and cook for about 7 minutes, until nicely browned on all sides. Transfer the lamb to a slow cooker. Add the stock to the pan and scrape up any brown bits, then pour over the lamb. Add the onions, carrots, tomatoes, ginger, garlic, cumin, cinnamon, and cayenne to the cooker. Cook on the high setting for 4 hours (or the low setting for 8), until the lamb is falling apart.

- Fifteen minutes before serving, stir in the chickpeas and raisins. Discard the cinnamon stick if using. Taste and adjust seasoning with salt and black pepper. Serve the tagine over the couscous and garnish with cilantro.

Makes 8 servings

Per Serving
$2.85
440 calories
25 g fat
(10 g saturated)
460 mg sodium

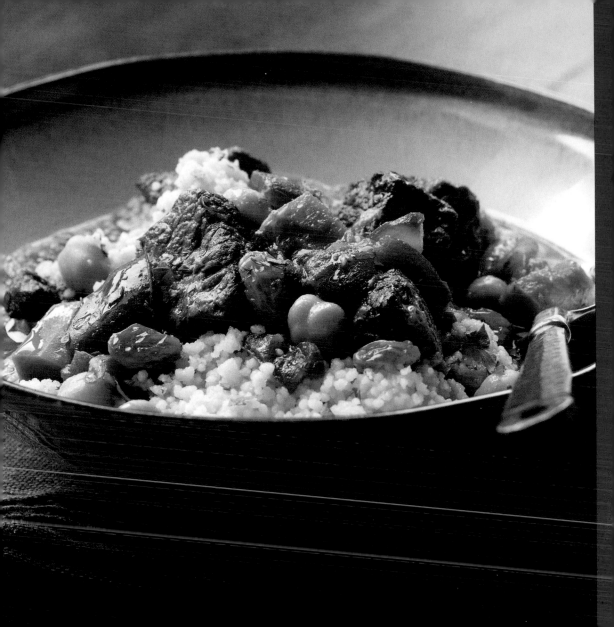

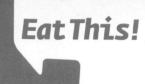

Kung Pao Chicken

What makes a stir-fry so incredibly comforting? We think that it is knowing that after a long, difficult day, a lean, flavor-packed meal can be prepared in a single pan in under 10 minutes for under $10. A real kung pao kicks like a karate kid, loaded with dried chiles that imbue the mash-up with a capsaicin glow. But in most versions across the restaurant and takeout spectrum, the heat takes a backseat to Chinese-American food's more dominant flavor profile: fat plus salt. This one puts heat back in the driver's seat.

You'll Need:

- 1 lb boneless, skinless chicken thighs, diced
- ¼ cup rice wine or sherry
- ¼ cup low-sodium chicken stock
- 2 Tbsp soy sauce
- 1 Tbsp balsamic vinegar
- ½ Tbsp sugar
- 1 tsp cornstarch
- 1 tsp sriracha or other Asian chili sauce
- 1 Tbsp peanut or canola oil
- 4 dried red chiles (or 1 tsp red pepper flakes)
- 4 scallions, chopped, white and green parts separated
- 3 cloves garlic, minced
- 1 Tbsp minced fresh ginger
- 1 large zucchini, diced
- 1 red bell pepper, diced
- ¼ cup roasted peanuts

You can adjust the heat to suit your own spice tolerance. Four chiles represents a medium-spicy kung pao.

Per Serving
$1.96
290 calories
13 g fat
(2 g saturated)
670 mg sodium

How to Make It:

- Combine the chicken, rice wine, stock, soy sauce, balsamic, sugar, cornstarch, and sriracha in a large bowl. Cover and marinate for 30 minutes, or up to 2 hours in the fridge.

- Heat the oil in a wok over medium-high heat. Add the chiles, scallion white parts, garlic, and ginger and stir-fry for 30 seconds, until fragrant but not browned. Add the zucchini and bell pepper and continue cooking, using a metal spatula to keep the ingredients in near-constant motion, for about 3 minutes, until the vegetables are lightly browned.

- Remove the chicken from the marinade and add to the wok, stir-frying for about 3 minutes, until lightly browned on the outside. Add the marinade and peanuts and cook for 3 minutes longer, until the liquid comes to a boil and begins to thicken and cling to the chicken and vegetables. Stir in the scallion greens and serve over a small scoop of steamed brown rice, if you like.

Makes 4 servings

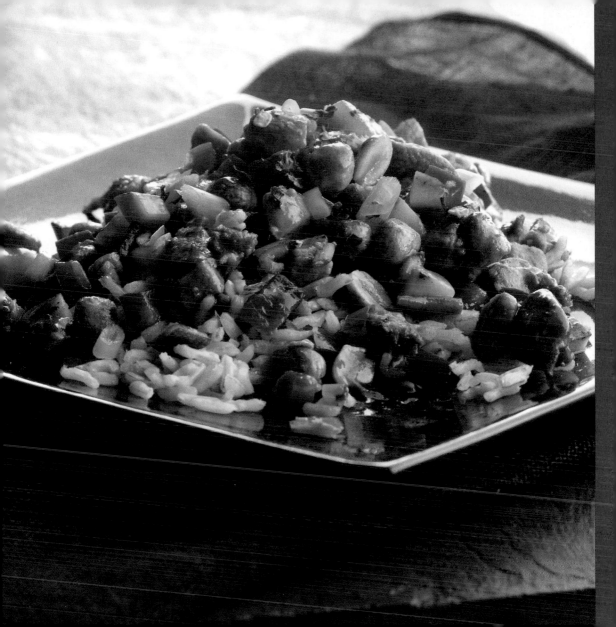

Chicken Tikka Masala

So dense is the Indian population and so ubiquitous their imprint on the country that many call tikka masala the national dish of England. It takes many years to master the complex spice art at the heart of Indian cuisine, but tikka masala is the perfect beginner's dish—light on ingredients and relatively mild in flavor. Tikka masala normally involves a heavy hand with both butter and cream, but we found that the combination of Greek yogurt and half-and-half gives you the same velvety texture for a fraction of the calories.

You'll Need:

- 4 cloves garlic, peeled
- 1" piece fresh ginger, peeled and roughly chopped
- 1 tsp cumin
- 1 tsp ground coriander
- ½ tsp ground cardamom
- ¾ tsp salt
- ½ tsp black pepper
- 1 cup 2% Greek yogurt
- 1 lb boneless, skinless chicken thighs
- ½ Tbsp olive oil
- 1 can (28 oz) crushed tomatoes
- ¼ cup half-and-half

How to Make It:

- Combine the garlic, ginger, cumin, coriander, cardamom, salt, and pepper in a mixing bowl. Spoon half of the mixture into a sealable plastic bag, along with ½ cup of the yogurt and the chicken. Squeeze the air out of the bag, seal, and massage the contents to evenly distribute. Refrigerate for at least 1 hour or up to 8 hours.
- Preheat the broiler.
- Heat the oil in a large saucepan or sauté pan over medium heat. Add the remaining ginger-spice mixture and sauté for about 3 minutes, until the ginger is soft. Add the tomatoes and simmer for 10 minutes. Turn the heat down to low and stir in the remaining ½ cup yogurt and the half-and-half and simmer while you broil the chicken.
- Remove the chicken from the bag and use paper towels to wipe the marinade from the chicken. Spread the chicken on a baking sheet and place directly underneath the broiler. Broil for about 2 minutes, until the top sides are nicely browned. Flip the chicken and broil for 2 minutes more. Rest for a few minutes, then chop into large pieces and add to the simmering tomato sauce. Simmer for 5 minutes, until the chicken is cooked through. Serve over steamed rice.

Makes 4 servings

Per Serving
$1.71
260 calories
8 g fat
(3 g saturated)
780 mg sodium

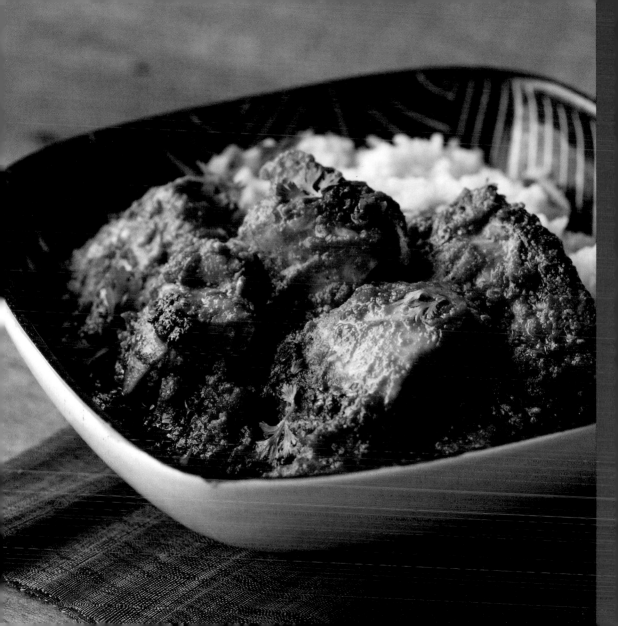

CHAPTER 11

VEGETABLE SIDES

America's Worst VEGETABLE SIDES

WORST BASIC VEGETABLE
Cheesecake Factory's Sautéed Spinach

270 calories
N/A g fat (13 g saturated)
907 mg sodium
Price: $4.95

Even spinach, arguably the most nutritious veggie on the planet, doesn't stand a chance when in the Cheesecake Factory's greasy grip. "Sautéed" is restaurant code for "soaked in butter," which is why you're looking at a leafy green with more than a day's worth of saturated fat— a pretty steep price to pay for an indulgent side, and absolute blasphemy for a scoop of produce. There are much safer ways to make your veggies go down smoothly, and they start in your home kitchen.

Eat This Instead!
Garlic-Lemon Spinach
(page 312)

80 calories
4 g fat (0.5 g saturated)
280 mg sodium
Cost per serving: $1.40
Save! 190 calories and $3.55!

568 calories

Ruby Tuesday's spud missile packs more calories than any recipe in this book.

Boston Market's Sweet Potato Casserole

450 calories
12 g fat (3 g saturated)
210 mg sodium
Price: $2.29

One of the main benefits of opting for sweet potatoes over standard spuds is that they cause less dramatic blood sugar spikes, a nutritional virtue that Boston Market completely nullifies by loading its yams with 15 (!) teaspoons of sugar. Thanks in part to a sweet streusel topping and a boatload of marshmallows, sugar shows up a total of seven times on this casserole's ingredients list, making it a dessert in disguise. And speaking of ingredients, this starchy side has far too many—a risk you take whenever you dine outside your own four walls.

Eat This Instead!
Yukon Gold & Sweet Potato Gratin (page 308)

210 calories
7 g fat (4.5 g saturated)
180 mg sodium
Cost per serving: $1.24
Save! 240 calories and $1.05!

Cheesecake Factory's Mashed Potatoes

470 calories
N/A g fat (21 g saturated)
703 mg sodium
Price: $4.95

Ordering mashed potatoes is risky business. Depending on how much butter and cream the restaurant chooses to stuff in its spuds, you could be getting the healthiest taters on the menu, or a starchy side, like this CF version, with more than a day's saturated fat and more calories than a large order of McDonald's french fries. That's no small potatoes, so if you want to avoid playing dietary Russian roulette, smash your spuds in the safety of your own home kitchen.

Eat This Instead!
Roasted Garlic Mashed Potatoes (page 302)

170 calories
5 g fat (3 g saturated)
270 mg sodium
Cost per serving: $0.61
Save! 300 calories and $4.34!

Ruby Tuesday's Loaded Baked Potato

562 calories
27 g fat (14 g saturated)
1,519 mg sodium
Price: $3.69

Not even baked potatoes are safe in the restaurant world. Chains get fancy with their taters to entice diners to drop more cash on a supposedly superior side, but the only benefit you'll get from topping your potato with butter, sour cream, bacon, and cheese is a protruding gut. Want to get fancy with the potato? Try a scoop of salsa.

Eat This Instead!
Twice Baked Potatoes (page 306)

200 calories
10 g fat (4 g saturated)
450 mg sodium
Cost per serving: $1.18
Save! 362 calories and $2.51!

T.G.I. Friday's Loaded Fries (with ranch dressing)

1,110 calories
71 g fat (22 g saturated)
3,000 mg sodium
Price: $2.99

Haven't the folks at Friday's heard that double dipping is frowned upon? These greasy potato sticks get not one, but two oil baths—a trip to the deep fryer and an extra dousing of oil to ensure the Parmesan sticks to the spuds—which is why they come with an entrée-worthy calorie count. If you want more slimming, satisfying fries, you're better off being left to your own device—the oven, that is.

Eat This Instead!
Crispy Oven-Baked Fries (page 298)

190 calories
8 g fat (1.5 g saturated)
240 mg sodium
Cost per serving: $0.57
Save! 920 calories and $2.42!

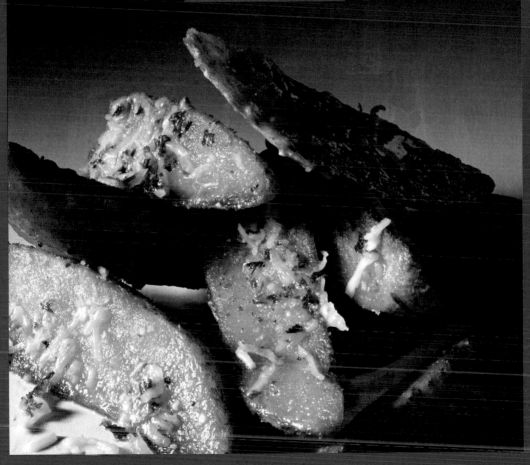

660 calories

Friday's fried potato wedges pack more calories than 4 Taco Bell Fresco beef tacos.

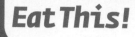

Crispy Oven-Baked Fries

Crispy baked fries: for so many years an oxymoron, now just 40 minutes away. The key here is washing the surface starch from the potatoes before baking, which helps encourage surface browning and crisping. The rosemary and Parmesan are nice touches, but the real star of this show is the spud itself.

You'll Need:

- 2 medium russet potatoes
- 2 Tbsp canola oil
- Salt to taste
- 2 cloves garlic, very finely minced
- 1 tsp fresh rosemary leaves
- ¼ cup grated Parmesan

How to Make It:

- Preheat the oven to 425°F.
- Peel the potatoes and cut into ¼-inch fries (about twice the thickness of standard fast-food fries). Soak in warm water for at least 15 minutes before cooking.
- Drain the potatoes and dry thoroughly.
- Combine the fries and the oil in a mixing bowl and toss until they're evenly coated.
- Season thoroughly with salt. Spread the fries out on a large baking sheet, being careful they don't overlap. Bake for 30 minutes, until the fries are just tender and lightly browned on the outside.
- Sprinkle with the garlic, rosemary, and Parmesan and return to the oven for another 10 minutes, until the cheese is melted and the garlic lightly browned.

Makes 4 servings

Per Serving
$0.57
190 calories
8 g fat
(1.5 g saturated)
240 mg sodium

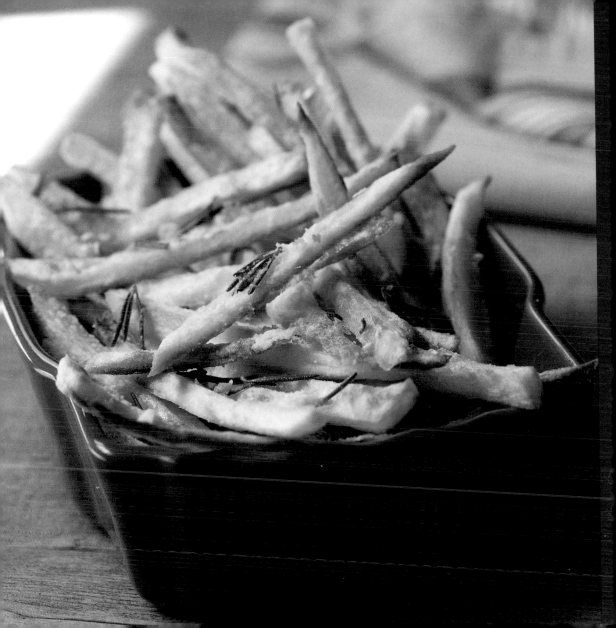

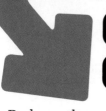

Eat This!

Green Bean Casserole

Perhaps the most famous back-of-the-box recipe ever, this home-cooked classic was invented in 1955 by the Campbell Soup Company, an ingenious way to get consumers to buy their Cream of Mushroom soup when items like fresh mushrooms and green beans were tough to come by. Those days, of course, are long gone, and the casserole is badly in need of an update. This version stays true to the original flavors (onions, mushrooms, green beans bound in a creamy sauce), but uses fresh ingredients to create something with texture, flavor, and nutrition far exceeding the original.

You'll Need:

Salt

- 1 lb green beans
- 1 Tbsp butter
- 1 red onion, thinly sliced
- 2 cloves garlic, minced
- 6 oz cremini mushrooms, sliced
- 2 Tbsp flour
- 1 cup low-sodium beef or chicken stock
- 1 cup 2% milk

Black pepper to taste

- ½ cup panko bread crumbs, tossed with 1 Tbsp olive oil

How to Make It:

- ● Bring a large pot of water to a boil. Season with salt and cook the green beans for about 3 minutes, until crisp-tender. Drain and run cold water over the beans to help stop the cooking.

- ● Preheat the oven to 475°F.

- ● Heat the butter in a large skillet over medium heat. Add the onions and garlic and cook for about 5 minutes, until the onions are very soft and translucent. Add the mushrooms and cook for about 5 minutes, until lightly browned. Stir in the flour and cook for 1 minute, then add the stock and milk, whisking to help prevent lumps from forming. Add the green beans and simmer for about 3 minutes, until the sauce thickens and clings to the vegetables. Season to taste with salt and black pepper.

- ● Pour the green beans into an 8" × 8" casserole dish and top with the bread crumbs. Place on the middle rack and bake for 8 to 10 minutes, until the bread crumbs are golden brown.

Makes 6 servings

Per Serving
$1.08
110 calories
2.5 g fat
(1.5 g saturated)
310 mg sodium

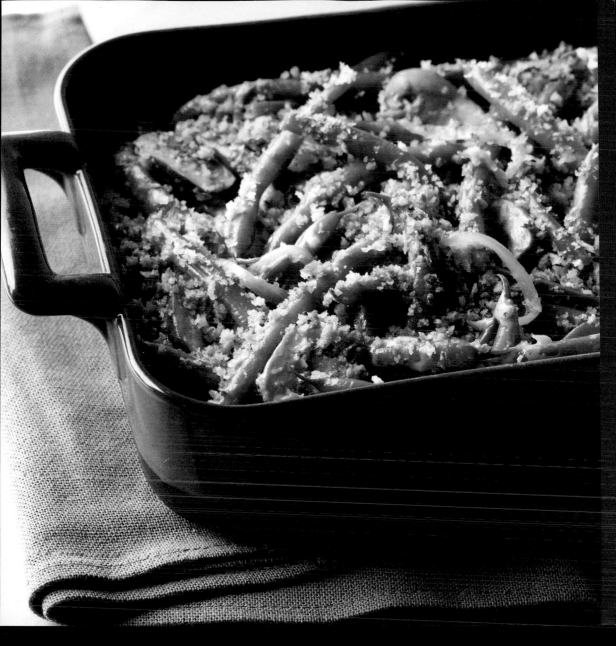

Roasted Garlic Mashed Potatoes

Everyone needs a great mashed potato recipe, and this is a perfect place to start: creamy and rich, but made with 2% milk and just a bit of butter. A potato ricer helps create smooth, fluffy mashed potatoes, but a potato masher or even a few active forks will work in a pinch.

You'll Need:

2 lbs Yukon gold potatoes, peeled and quartered

Salt to taste

1 cup 2% milk

Roasted Garlic (page 321)

2 Tbsp butter

Black pepper to taste

Chopped fresh chives or minced rosemary (optional)

How to Make It:

- Fill a large saucepan with water and add the potatoes. Season with a few pinches of salt and bring to a boil. Cook for about 20 minutes, until the potatoes are just tender. Drain.

- While the potatoes cook, combine the milk and garlic in a small saucepan and bring to a simmer. Use a fork or a potato masher to mash the garlic into the milk. Keep warm until the potatoes are cooked.

- If you have a potato ricer, rice the drained potatoes into a large bowl. If not, mash them with a potato masher or the largest forks you can find. Add the butter to the potatoes and continue mashing. Next, stir in the milk, one large spoonful at a time, using a wooden spoon to help whip the liquid into the potatoes (this will create a smoother, more stable emulsion).

- Season with salt and black pepper and stir in any herbs you may be using.

Makes 6 servings

Per Serving
$0.61
170 calories
5 g fat
(3 g saturated)
270 mg sodium

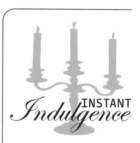

Indulgence **INSTANT**

Trick out your mashed potatoes with any of these extras:

- Artichoke hearts, lemon zest, and grated Parmesan
- Crumbled bacon, sharp Cheddar, and minced scallions
- Sun-dried tomatoes, chopped olives, and crumbled goat cheese or feta
- Caramelized onions and grated horseradish

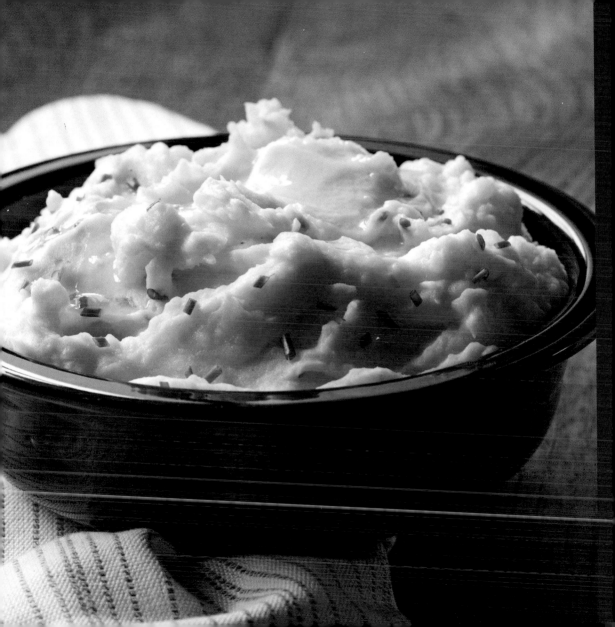

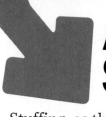

Eat This!

Apple-Sausage Stuffing

Stuffing, as the name implies, was once invariably cooked inside the bird, where rendered turkey juices would transform it into a savory mush. Delicious, to be sure, but lacking in texture and loaded with calories. These days, stuffing is most often baked on its own, which gives you full control over the final taste, texture, and nutritional profile, but also means you need to punch up the flavors. We turn to the combination of sausage, tart apples, and fresh sage, which effortlessly converts a normal stuffing into something extraordinary—equally good with Garlic-Rosemary Roast Beef (page 208), Bourbon-Glazed Ham (page 214), or a giant holiday bird (page 186).

You'll Need:

1 tsp olive oil

2 links turkey sausage, preferably apple, casings removed

1 medium onion, diced

2 stalks celery, diced

1 Granny Smith apple, cored, peeled, and diced

½ cup dried cranberries

2 cloves garlic, minced

5 cups cubed bread from a sturdy loaf or baguette, preferably whole wheat

Slightly stale bread works best. If the bread is fresh, place in a 350°F oven for 10 minutes before using.

10–12 leaves fresh sage, chopped

1½ cups low-sodium chicken stock

1 egg, beaten

Salt and black pepper to taste

2 Tbsp cold butter, diced

How to Make It:

● Heat the olive oil in a large skillet over medium heat. Add the sausage, onion, celery, apple, cranberries, and garlic and sauté for about 10 minutes, until the vegetables are soft and the sausage is just cooked through.

● Combine the bread, sausage-vegetable mixture, sage, stock, and egg in a large mixing bowl. Toss to evenly coat the stuffing with the liquid. Season with a few pinches of salt and black pepper. Place in a 13" x 9" casserole dish and dot with the butter.

● Bake, uncovered, for about 40 minutes, until the top of the stuffing is nicely browned and crunchy.

Makes 6 to 8 servings.

Per Serving
$1.37
160 calories
7 g fat
(2.5 g saturated)
290 mg sodium

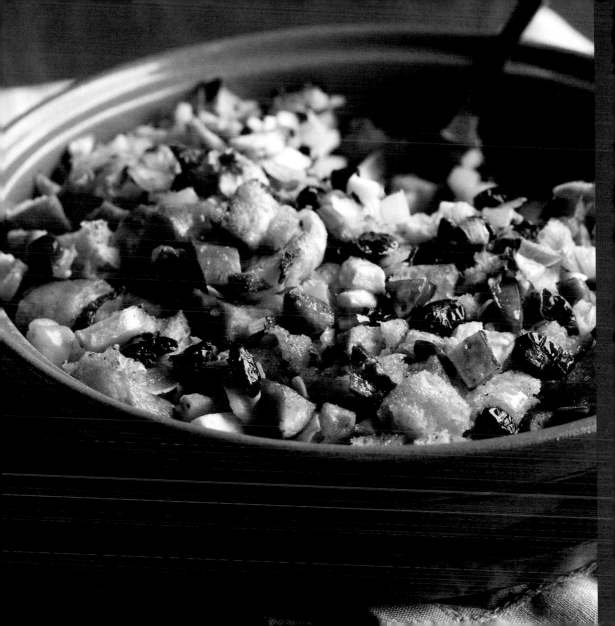

Twice-Baked Potatoes

"Twice baked" normally means twice as caloric, but we keep matters in control by employing milk and yogurt to enrich these potatoes. Of course, a little bit of cheese and bacon go a long way toward giving the spuds the indulgent feel they demand. Perfect with a grilled steak, but these could also double as potato skins for an appetizer or snack during the ballgame.

You'll Need:

2 **medium russet potatoes**

Olive oil for coating the potatoes

4 **strips bacon, cooked and crumbled**

½ **cup 2% milk**

1 **Tbsp butter**

2 **Tbsp Greek yogurt**

½ **cup chopped scallions (green parts only)**

½ **cup shredded sharp Cheddar cheese**

Tabasco to taste

Salt and black pepper to taste

How to Make It:

- Preheat the oven to 375°F. Prick the potatoes all over with a fork, then rub with a light layer of oil. Place on the middle rack of the oven and bake for about 40 minutes, until tender all the way through. Increase the oven temperature to 450°F.

- When the potatoes have cooled slightly, cut them in half lengthwise and carefully scoop out the flesh, being careful not to tear the skins. Combine the potato flesh in a mixing bowl with the bacon, milk, butter, yogurt, scallions, about three-fourths of the cheese, Tabasco, and salt and pepper. Mix thoroughly, then divide among the potato skins. Top with the remaining cheese. Return to the oven and bake for 7 to 10 minutes, until browned on top.

Makes 4 servings

Cook the bacon for 15 minutes on a baking sheet alongside the potatoes.

Per Serving
$1.18
200 calories
10 g fat
(4 g saturated)
450 mg sodium

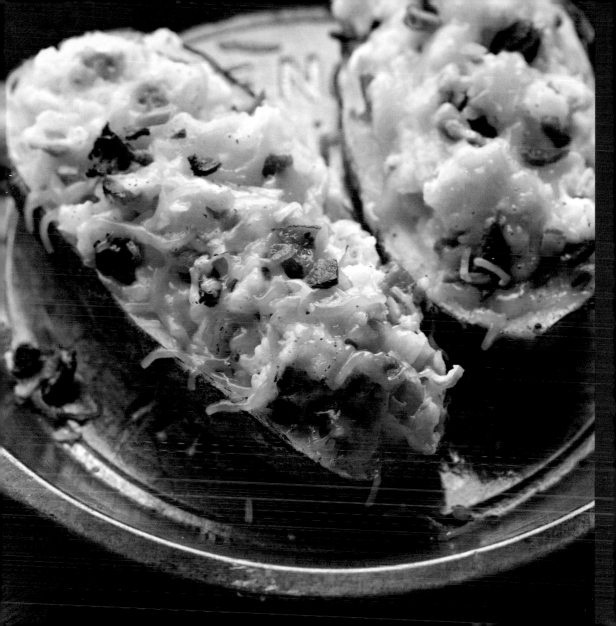

Yukon Gold & Sweet Potato Gratin

The basic idea behind a gratin is to turn the potato into a vessel for heavy cream and butter, which explains why a side portion of a restaurant gratin could have more calories than the entrée it accompanies. We slim our version down by trading in milk for the traditional cream and buffering the normal potatoes with nutrient-dense, fiber-loaded sweet potatoes. Try this with a roasted chicken, a grilled steak, or your next Thanksgiving turkey.

You'll Need:

2 Tbsp butter

2 Tbsp flour

2 cups 2% milk

Pinch nutmeg

2 medium Yukon gold potatoes, peeled and sliced into ⅛"-thick slices

2 medium sweet potatoes, peeled and sliced into ⅛"-thick slices

Salt and black pepper to taste

½ cup grated Gruyère or other Swiss cheese

Fresh chopped rosemary for garnish (optional)

How to Make It:

● Preheat the oven to 375°F.

● Melt the butter in a medium saucepan over medium heat. Stir in the flour and cook, stirring, for 1 minute to help eliminate a bit of that raw flour taste. Slowly add the milk, whisking to help prevent lumps from forming. Simmer the béchamel for 5 minutes, until it begins to thicken to the consistency of heavy cream. Season with the nutmeg.

● Layer the potatoes in an overlapping pattern in the bottom of a 10" cast-iron skillet or 8" x 8" baking dish, alternating between regular and sweet potatoes and seasoning each layer with salt and black pepper. (You should have enough potatoes to make a 4-layer gratin.) Pour over the béchamel, then top with the grated cheese.

● Cover with foil and bake for 20 minutes. Increase the temperature to 450°F. Remove the foil and continue baking for about 20 minutes, until the surface of the gratin is nicely browned all over.

Makes 6 servings

Per Serving
$1.24
210 calories
7 g fat
(4.5 g saturated)
180 mg sodium

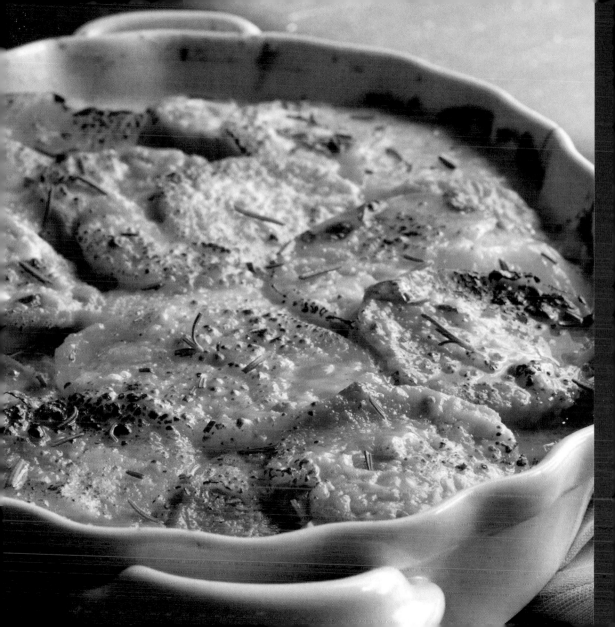

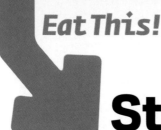

Eat This!

Stuffed Tomatoes

Just 2 minutes of prep work and 20 minutes of cooking turn normal tomatoes into something memorable: sweet, creamy, crunchy, and imbued with faint whispers of garlic and fresh basil. If you want to take these over the top, try wrapping each tomato with a slice of prosciutto before baking. Pork or not, these are a perfect partner for Steaks with Red Wine Sauce (page 222) or Smothered Pork Chops (page 210).

You'll Need:

- 4 medium beefsteak or other round tomatoes
- 1 cup panko bread crumbs
- ½ cup fresh goat cheese or feta
- ¼ cup chopped fresh basil
- 1 Tbsp olive oil
- 2 tsp finely minced garlic

Salt and black pepper to taste

How to Make It:

- Preheat the oven to 400°F.
- Cut the tops off the tomatoes and use a spoon to scoop out the core and seeds and discard. In a mixing bowl, combine the bread crumbs, cheese, basil, olive oil, and garlic and season with salt and black pepper. Stuff the tomatoes with the mixture.
- Place the tomatoes in a baking dish and bake for about 20 minutes, until the bread crumbs are golden brown and the tomatoes are lightly caramelized.

Makes 4 servings

Per Serving
$1.46
160 calories
8 g fat
(3.5 g saturated)
360 mg sodium

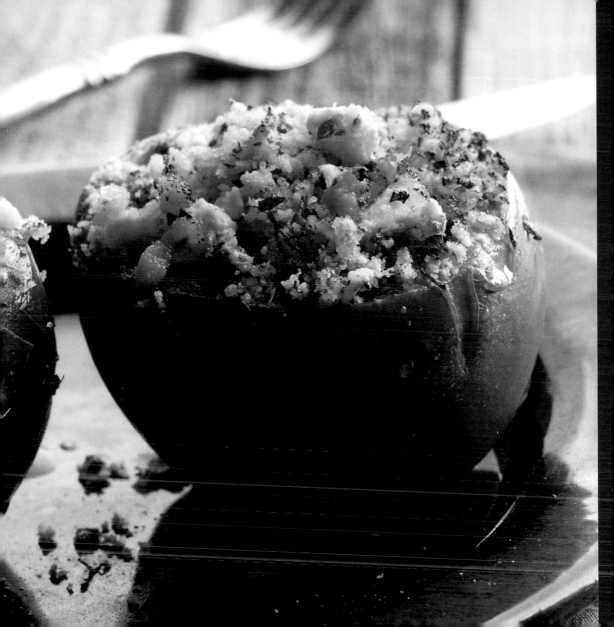

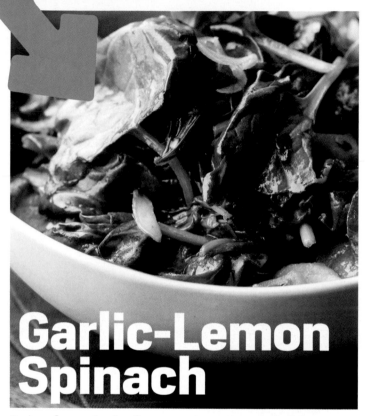

Eat This!

Garlic-Lemon Spinach

You'll Need:

1 Tbsp olive oil

3 cloves garlic, thinly sliced

Pinch red pepper flakes

2 bunches spinach, stems removed, washed and dried

Juice of 1 lemon

Salt and black pepper to taste

How to Make It:

● Heat the olive oil in a large sauté or saucepan over medium-low heat. Add the garlic and red pepper flakes and cook gently for about 3 minutes, until the garlic is lightly browned. Add the spinach and cook, moving the uncooked spinach to the bottom of the pan with tongs, for about 5 minutes, until fully wilted. Drain off any excess water from the bottom of the pan. Stir in the lemon juice and season to taste with salt and black pepper.

Makes 4 servings

Spinach got its bad reputation among finicky eaters because most people have had to endure plates of plain boiled or steamed greens, which taste like nothing but chlorophyll. This version, rich with garlic- and red pepper—infused olive oil, will convert the most closed-minded skeptics.

Per Serving
$1.40
80 calories
4 g fat
(0.5 g saturated)
280 mg sodium

Potato Salad

This version is about as classic as potato salad gets, except for the fact that we resist the urge to drown the vegetables in a viscous sea of mayo. Instead, the mayo is bolstered with Dijon and a tangy shot of vinegar. The result: a healthier potato salad that still tastes like the picnic classic we all adore.

You'll Need:

3 lbs red potatoes, all similar in size

Salt and black pepper to taste

2 stalks celery, chopped

¼ cup chopped pickles (preferably gherkins or cornichons)

1 small red onion, chopped

2 Tbsp Dijon mustard

½ cup mayonnaise

2 Tbsp white wine vinegar

3 hard-boiled eggs, chopped

Smoked paprika (optional)

How to Make It:

- Place the potatoes in a large pot and fill with enough cold water to easily cover. Season the water with 1 teaspoon salt and bring to a boil. Cook the potatoes until tender all the way through (the tip of a paring knife inserted into a potato will meet little resistance). Drain.

- When cool enough to handle, chop the potatoes into ¾" pieces. Place in a large bowl and add the celery, pickles, onion, mustard, mayonnaise, vinegar, and eggs. Toss to coat. Season with salt and pepper and sprinkle with the paprika (if using).

Makes 10 servings

Per Serving
$0.92
190 calories
10 g fat
(2 g saturated)
320 mg sodium

Smoky Baked Beans

Baked beans, both the type that come in cans and those that come from the kitchens of barbecue shacks, are usually one step away from candy, bombarded as they are with brown sugar, molasses, and honey. Too bad, since beans really are A-list eats. To preserve their health status and maximize deliciousness, we mitigate the sugar surge and build flavor instead with a few of our all-time favorite foods: cayenne, beer, and bacon.

You'll Need:

4 strips bacon, chopped into small pieces

1 medium onion, minced

2 cloves garlic, minced

2 cans (16 oz each) pinto beans, rinsed and drained

1 cup dark beer

¼ cup ketchup

1 Tbsp chili powder

1 Tbsp brown sugar

Pinch of cayenne pepper

How to Make It:

- Heat a large pot or saucepan over medium heat. Add the bacon and cook until it's just turning crispy, 3 to 5 minutes. Add the onion and garlic and sauté until translucent, another 3 minutes. Stir in the beans, beer, ketchup, chili powder, brown sugar, and cayenne. Simmer until the sauce thickens and clings to the beans, about 15 minutes.

Makes 6 servings

Per Serving
$0.81
170 calories
3 g fat
(1 g saturated)
570 mg sodium

Eat This!

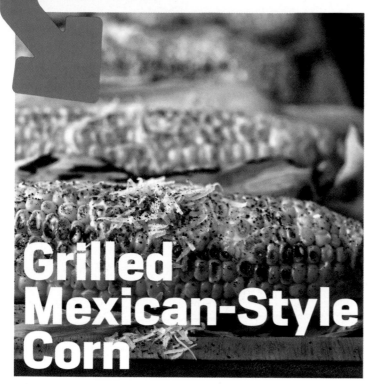

Grilled Mexican-Style Corn

You'll Need:

4 ears of corn, husked

1 tsp salt

2 Tbsp mayonnaise

Juice of 1 lime

½ Tbsp chili powder

Finely grated Parmesan

How to Make It:

- Heat a grill until hot. While the grill is warming up, bring a pot of water to a boil. Add the corn and salt. Boil for 5 to 7 minutes, until the corn until slightly tender, but not cooked all the way through. Drain the corn and transfer to the grill; lightly char the kernels.

- Mix the mayonnaise and lime juice. Remove the corn from the grill, paint with a bit of the citrus mayonnaise, then dust with chili powder and Parmesan.

Makes 4 servings

This is how corn is served on the streets of Mexico, robed in a thin sheen of mayo (instead of butter) and topped with a sprinkling of chili powder and cheese. If you want to cut the calories, lime juice and chili powder alone offer a vast improvement over standard boiled corn—but once you try the full package, you'll have a hard time eating it any other way.

Per Serving
$0.64
210 calories
9 g fat
(2 g saturated)
430 mg sodium

Cole Slaw

Crunchy, cool, and suffused with vinegar tang, this slaw has nothing to do with those soupy, mayo-drenched, oversweetened versions you find in most supermarket deli cases. Great as a side, but also perfect for topping sandwiches.

You'll Need:

- 2 Tbsp Dijon mustard
- 2 Tbsp mayonnaise
- 2 Tbsp vinegar (red wine, white wine, or cider)
- 2 Tbsp canola oil

Salt and black pepper to taste

- ½ head green cabbage, very thinly sliced
- ½ head red cabbage, very thinly sliced
- 3 carrots, cut into thin strips
- 1 tsp fennel seeds

How to Make It:

- Mix the mustard, mayonnaise, and vinegar in a bowl. Slowly whisk in the oil. Season with salt and pepper.
- Combine the cabbages, carrots, fennel seeds, and dressing in a large bowl. Toss so that everything is evenly coated and season with more salt and pepper.

Makes 6 servings

Per Serving
$0.78
130 calories
8 g fat
(1 g saturated)
200 mg sodium

Parmesan-Roasted Broccoli

This simple roasting technique can be applied to any of a dozen different vegetables: asparagus, cauliflower, Brussels sprouts, red potatoes. Of course, the times will vary depending on the vegetable of choice (asparagus will be done in less than 10 minutes; potatoes will take closer to 30), but the results are uniformly satisfying.

You'll Need:

- 1 head broccoli, cut into florets, bottom part of the stem removed
- 1 Tbsp olive oil

Salt and black pepper to taste

- ¼ cup grated Parmesan cheese

How to Make It:

- Preheat the oven to 450°F. Toss the broccoli with the olive oil, salt, and pepper and spread out evenly on a baking sheet. Roast in the oven until the broccoli is tender and lightly browned, about 12 minutes. Remove from the oven, toss with the cheese, and serve.

Makes 4 servings

Per Serving
$0.91
100 calories
5 g fat
(1.5 g saturated)
220 mg sodium

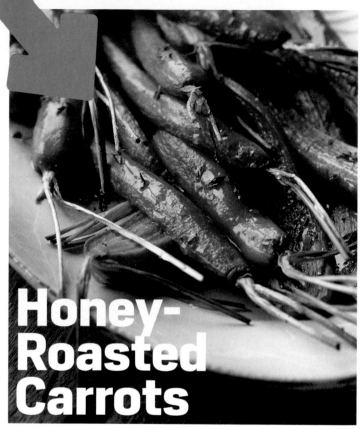

Honey-Roasted Carrots

The difference between boring vegetables and exciting ones sometimes boils down to one or two ingredients. Here, honey and thyme transform otherwise pedestrian carrots into something crave worthy.

You'll Need:

- 1 bunch carrots, tops trimmed, peeled, and halved
- 1 Tbsp olive oil
- 1 Tbsp fresh thyme (or ½ tsp dried thyme)

Salt and black pepper to taste

- 2 Tbsp honey

How to Make It:

- Preheat the oven 425°F.
- Toss the carrots with the olive oil and thyme and season with salt and pepper. Place on a baking sheet and roast on the middle rack of the oven for about 15 minutes, until the carrots are soft and just beginning to brown. Drizzle with the honey and use tongs to toss the carrots so that they're evenly coated. Return to the oven and roast for about 10 minutes longer, until the honey caramelizes and the surface of the carrots turns a deep brown color.

Makes 4 servings

Per Serving
$0.72
110 calories
3.5 g fat
(0.5 g saturated)
220 mg sodium

Smoked Paprika Potato Chips

These chips aren't just considerably better for you than the standard supermarket fried variety, they're also about three times as delicious, thanks to the fresh potato flavor and a smoky touch from paprika. Eat them as a snack, or serve alongside a grilled steak or a burger.

You'll Need:

- 1 large russet potato
- 2 Tbsp olive oil
- 1 tsp smoked paprika

Salt and black pepper to taste

How to Make It:

- Preheat the oven to 350°F. Peel the potato and slice as thinly and uniformly as possible. (If you have a kitchen mandoline, now's the time to use it.)
- Soak the potato slices for at least 5 minutes in cold water. Drain and pat dry, then toss in a bowl with the olive oil, paprika, salt, and pepper.
- Lay the potatoes out on an oiled baking sheet. (The slices can overlap.) Bake until the potatoes are golden brown and crunchy, about 30 minutes.

Makes 4 servings

Per Serving
$0.38
130 calories
7 g fat
(1 g saturated)
150 mg sodium

Brussels & Bacon

Brussels sprouts are the type of food that strikes horror in the hearts of picky eaters. We promise, the smoke of the bacon, the heat of the red pepper flakes, and the crunch of the almonds will win over even the most stubborn veggie-phobe.

You'll Need:

- 4 strips bacon, chopped into small pieces
- 2 cloves garlic, peeled
- 1 tsp red pepper flakes
- 1 lb Brussels sprouts, bottoms trimmed, cut in half

Salt to taste

- 2 Tbsp sliced almonds

Black pepper to taste

How to Make It:

- Heat a large skillet or sauté pan over medium heat. Add the bacon and cook until crispy, about 5 minutes. Remove to a plate lined with paper towels. Discard all but 1 tablespoon of the rendered bacon fat.
- Add the garlic, pepper flakes, Brussels sprouts, and a pinch of salt to the skillet. Sauté until the sprouts are lightly browned on the outside and tender—but still firm—throughout, 10 to 12 minutes. Add the almonds and sauté for another minute or two. Season with salt and pepper.

Makes 4 servings

Per Serving
$0.64
210 calories
9 g fat
(2 g saturated)
430 mg sodium

317

Secret WEAPONS

It always helps to have a few secret weapons up your sleeve. These 10 sauces, salsas, and rubs hail from all over the world, but they share one thing in common: They bring maximum flavor impact with minimum effort. Have at least a few of them in the fridge at all times and you can turn even the dullest meal into something memorable.

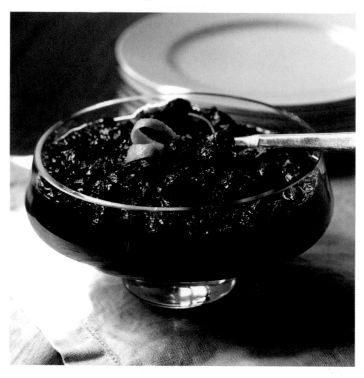

Orange-Cranberry Relish

Amazing with a Thanksgiving bird, of course, but also great with roast chicken or spread on sandwiches.

You'll Need:

    1 bag (12 oz) frozen cranberries

Zest and juice from 1 orange

    ⅓ cup sugar, plus more if needed

    1 tsp fresh grated ginger

How to Make It:

- Combine the cranberries, orange juice, sugar, and ginger in a saucepan set over medium heat. Simmer for 20 to 25 minutes, until the cranberries break down to form a thick sauce. Taste and adjust the sweetness with more sugar if necessary. Add the orange zest just before serving.

Makes about 15 servings

Chimichurri

Chimichurri, an herb-based sauce from Argentina, is used to adorn and enhance a variety of different dishes—grilled meats and fish above all. After some careful reflection, we've decided that chimi is pretty much the world's greatest condiment, turning mediocre food good and making good food great. Once you make it, you'll have a hard time not painting it on everything you come across: sandwiches, grilled vegetables, eggs.

You'll Need:

- 1 cup rough chopped parsley (about half a bunch)
- 1 clove garlic
- ½ tsp salt
- 2 Tbsp water
- 1½ Tbsp red wine vinegar
- ¼ cup oil
- ½ tsp sugar
- 1 Tbsp minced jalapeño

How to Make It:

- Combine all ingredients in a food processor and pulse until fully blended.

Makes roughly 1 cup; keeps in the refrigerator for up to one week

Classic Barbecue Sauce

Consider this your barbecue-sauce blueprint; from here, you can adjust with ingredients like honey, beer, hot sauce, or anything else that excites your taste buds.

You'll Need:

- 2 Tbsp butter
- 1 small onion, minced
- 1 cup ketchup
- 2 Tbsp brown sugar
- 2 Tbsp apple cider vinegar
- 1 Tbsp Worcestershire sauce
- ½ Tbsp dry mustard
- ⅓ tsp paprika (preferably smoked)
- ½ tsp garlic powder
- ⅛ tsp cayenne
- Black pepper to taste

How to Make It:

- In a medium saucepan, melt the butter over low heat. Add the onion and sauté until soft and translucent. Stir in the ketchup, brown sugar, vinegar, Worcestershire, mustard, paprika, garlic powder, cayenne, and a few pinches of black pepper. Simmer over low heat for 15 minutes until you have a thick, uniform sauce.

Makes about 1½ cups; keeps in the refrigerator for up to 2 weeks

Pico de Gallo

This chunky, fresh tomato salsa comes together with about 3 minutes' worth of knife work, yet it adds a complex trio of sweet, heat, and acid to everything from sandwiches to grilled fish.

You'll Need:

- 2 lbs Roma tomatoes, seeded and chopped
- 1 small red onion, diced
- 1 jalapeño pepper, seeded and minced
- ½ cup chopped cilantro
- Juice of 1 lime
- Salt to taste

How to Make It:

- Combine the tomatoes, onion, jalapeño, cilantro, and lime juice in a mixing bowl. Season with salt.

Makes about 3 cups; keeps for 3 days in the refrigerator

Pesto

You can buy perfectly fine pesto in the refrigerated section of most supermarkets (we like Cibo), but it will never taste as good as a homemade batch—which, by the way, takes all of 3 minutes to make. It works equally well as a marinade as it does for a post-grill dipping sauce. To keep it extra fresh and green, float a thin layer of oil on top of the pesto before refrigerating—the oil will keep the basil from oxidizing and turning dark. Try substituting arugula for the basil for a peppery alternative.

You'll Need:

- 2 cloves garlic, chopped
- 2 Tbsp pine nuts
- 3 cups fresh basil leaves
- ¼ cup grated Parmesan
- Salt and black pepper to taste
- ½ cup olive oil

How to Make It:

- Place the garlic, pine nuts, basil, and Parmesan, plus a few pinches of salt and pepper, in a food processor. Pulse until the basil is chopped. With the motor running, slowly drizzle in the olive oil until fully incorporated and a paste forms.

Makes about 1 cup; keeps for 2 weeks in the refrigerator

Magic Blackening Rub

Coat meat, fish, or vegetables with this potent blend of seasonings and cook over high heat until it transforms into a dark, savory crust.

You'll Need:

- 1 Tbsp paprika
- 1 Tbsp salt
- 2 tsp black pepper
- 2 tsp ground cumin
- 2 tsp garlic powder
- 2 tsp onion powder
- 1 tsp dried oregano
- ½ tsp cayenne pepper

How to Make It:

- Mix all of the spices together in a bowl or plastic storage container.

Makes about ⅓ cup; keeps in your spice cabinet for up to 2 months

Guacamole

Many American versions of guacamole include ingredients like cumin, sour cream, and (gasp!) mayo. But guac is really at its best with just a few carefully balanced ingredients: garlic, a good pinch of salt, and a squeeze of lemon or lime. And of course, perfectly ripe Hass avocados. Use that as your base; everything else— onion, jalapeño, cilantro, tomato— is just a bonus.

You'll Need:

- 2 cloves garlic, peeled
- Kosher salt to taste
- ¼ cup minced red onion
- 1 Tbsp minced jalapeño
- 2 ripe avocados, pitted and peeled
- Juice of 1 lemon or lime
- Chopped fresh cilantro (optional)

How to Make It:

- Use the side of a knife to smash the garlic against the cutting board. Finely mince the cloves, then apply a pinch of salt to the garlic and use the side of your knife to work the garlic into a paste. Scoop the garlic into a bowl, then add the onion, jalapeño, and avocados and mash until the avocados are puréed, but still slightly chunky. Stir in the lemon juice, cilantro (if using), and salt to taste.

Makes about 2 cups

Roasted Garlic

Raw garlic can be harsh and overpowering. Overcooked garlic can be acrid and off-putting. But slow-roasted garlic is like savory candy—sweet and inviting with its mellowed garlic flavor. Fold into mashed potatoes or salad dressings (especially Caesar) or simply spread on on a loaf of bread, top with a bit of Parmesan, and bake until brown for heroic garlic bread.

You'll Need:

- 1 head of garlic
- 1 Tbsp olive oil

How to Make It:

- Preheat the oven to 325°F. Separate the garlic cloves and peel them. Place in the center of a large piece of aluminum foil and drizzle with the oil. Fold the foil to enclose the garlic. Place on a baking sheet and bake for 35 to 40 minutes, until the garlic is soft enough to spread like warm butter. Transfer to a covered jar or container.

Store in the fridge for up to 2 weeks

Tomato Sauce

You won't find a simpler recipe in this book, but this bright, sweet, lightly acidic sauce is perfect for pizzas and topping dishes like Chicken Parm (page 188). For a real marinara, simmer this mix below in a saucepan with garlic and onions, then accentuate with flavor boosters like red pepper flakes or fresh basil.

You'll Need:

- 1 (28 oz) can whole peeled tomatoes, liquid discarded
- 1 Tbsp olive oil
- ½ tsp salt

How to Make It:

- Use your hands to lightly crush the tomatoes through your fingers (careful, juice can spray out). Stir in the oil and season with salt.

Makes about 2 cups

Romesco

This Catalan condiment is used throughout Spain as a dip for vegetables and a sauce for grilled meats and fish. It's at its best when served alongside lightly charred asparagus spears, tuna steaks, a few slices of sirloin, or some roasted potatoes.

You'll Need:

- 3 Tbsp olive oil
- 2 slices bread, torn into small pieces
- 2 Tbsp chopped almonds
- 2 cloves garlic, chopped
- 1 tsp smoked paprika
- ½ jar (12 oz) roasted red peppers
- 1 Tbsp red wine vinegar or sherry vinegar

Salt and black pepper to taste

How to Make It:

- Heat 1 tablespoon of the olive oil in a medium sauté pan set over medium heat. Add the bread crumbs, almonds, garlic, and paprika and sauté for about 5 minutes, until the bread is lightly golden and crunchy. Transfer to a blender and add the remaining 2 tablespoons olive oil, the red peppers, vinegar, and a sprinkle of salt and pepper; purée until smooth.

Makes about 2 cups

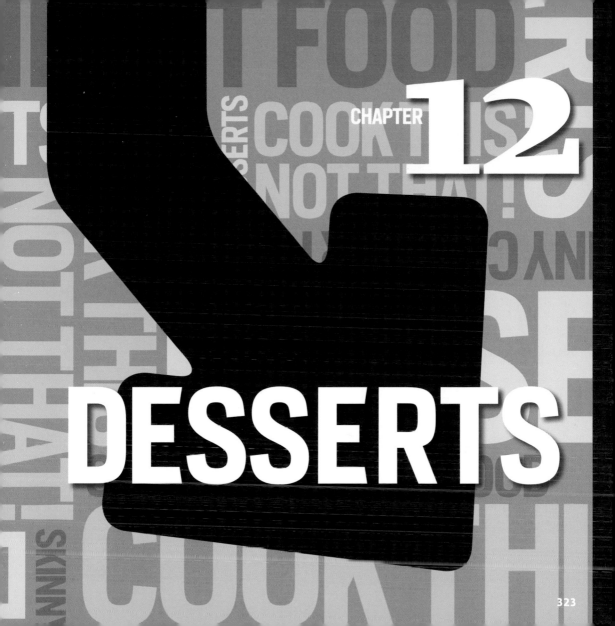

CHAPTER **12**

DESSERTS

America's Worst DESSERTS

WORST KEY LIME PIE
California Pizza Kitchen's Key Lime Pie (1 slice)

790 calories
44 g fat (25 g saturated)
94 g carbs
Price: $6.25

Key lime tends to be the bad seed of the fruit-pie lot, a fact owed to its rich, creamy filling and buttery graham cracker crust. And when it's prepared according to the more-is-more philosophy common at American chains like CPK, this

Southern classic can easily go from unruly to downright defiant. In our recipe, we teach you how to make a version of the citrusy treat that packs the perfect balance of rebellion and obedience. Mom would be so proud.

Eat This Instead!
Key Lime Pie (page 336)

330 calories
10 g fat (5 g saturated)
39 g sugars
Cost per serving: $1.34
Save! 460 calories and $4.91!

WORST CHEESECAKE
Cheesecake Factory's Wild Blueberry White Chocolate Cheesecake

990 calories
N/A g fat (44 g saturated)
98 g carbs
Price: $6.95

After filling up on the Factory's uber-fattening fare, we're surprised their patrons can even look at the cheesecake menu. But if you dare to sneak a peak, this is what you'll find: an array of

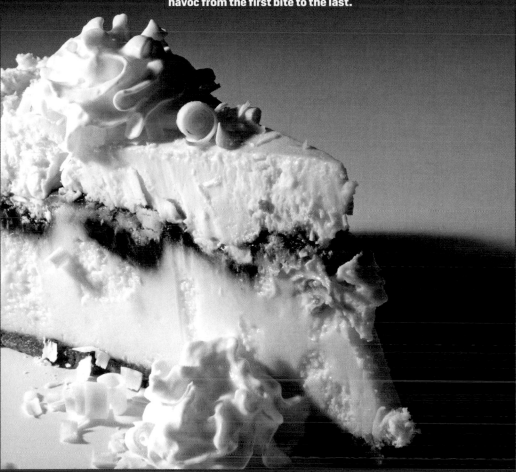

44 grams of saturated fat
Cheesecake Factory's namesake dessert proves the chain can cause havoc from the first bite to the last.

brick-sized slices all hovering around the 1,000-calorie mark. Depressing right? But don't worry, there's an antidote to your cheesecake blues: ricotta. Yep, the simple swap from cream cheese to ricotta makes for a cheesecake slice with fewer calories, more protein, and less fat. But since you won't find the Italian cheese in many chain kitchens, we brought you a delectable recipe that'll let you have your cheesecake and eat it, too.

Eat This Instead!
Ricotta Cheesecake
(page 332)
360 calories
19 g fat (8 g saturated)
40 g carbs
Cost per serving: $1.96
Save! 630 calories and $4.99!

WORST BROWNIE
Bob Evans's Peanut Butter Brownie Bites
1,024 calories
49 g fat (13 g saturated)
96 g sugars
Price: $4.00

"Bites" sounds more innocent than a full-blown brownie, but in this case, the modest word is nothing but a marketing ploy. What you have here is two of the chain's standard peanut butter brownies sliced up into smaller pieces. And by "standard," we mean "enormous." Restaurants consistently pump out bulging

baked goods that pack far more calories than their homemade counterparts, and when you consider that sweet treats also taste better warm out of your own oven, you really have no excuse for not donning that apron.

Eat This Instead!
Fudgy Brownies (page 334)
200 calories
12.5 g fat (6 g saturated)
16 g sugars
Cost per serving: $0.46
Save! 824 calories and $3.54!

WORST CHOCOLATE CAKE
Chili's Molten Chocolate Cake
1,150 calories
61 g fat (30 g saturated)
142 g carbs
Price: $6.29

A dome of moist chocolate cake erupting with gooey chocolate lava is every cocoa lover's fantasy, and though we don't make a habit of crushing dreams, we've gotta call this vicious volcano out. First off, there are more calories here than five Hershey's Milk Chocolate bars. Second, thanks in part to a crown of chocolate-smothered ice cream, this dessert houses 2½ days' worth of saturated fat. You can afford to eat a dessert like this a few times a year; the rest of the year, turn to our version—as rich and chocolaty as anything you'll

find in a restaurant, but with a third of the calories of Chili's version.

Eat This Instead!
Molten Chocolate Cake
(page 344)
320 calories
22 g fat (11 g saturated)
31 g carbs
Cost per serving: $1.20
Save! 830 calories and $5.09!

WORST BANANA DESSERT
Uno Chicago Grill's Bananas Foster
1,280 calories
64 g fat (36 g saturated)
129 g sugars
Price: $4.99

We don't know who Foster is, but he sure hates bananas. This New Orleans classic takes the nutritious yellow-peeled fruit, drowns it in butter, smothers it with sugar, douses it with rum, and sets it on fire. And as if this nutritional beating weren't bad enough, chains like Uno usually serve the dish in out-of-control portions, a move that, here, makes for a banana treat with more sugar than an entire carton of Ben & Jerry's Chunky Monkey ice cream. Bananas!

Eat This Instead!
Banana Pudding (page 330)
290 calories
7 g fat (2 g saturated)
36 g sugars
Cost per serving: $0.65
Save! 990 calories and $4.34!

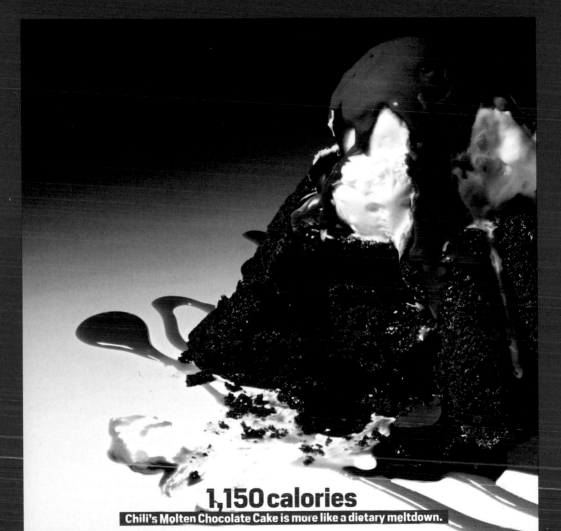

1,150 calories

Chili's Molten Chocolate Cake is more like a dietary meltdown.

Oatmeal-Chocolate Chip Cookies

The wonder of the oatmeal-chocolate chip cookie lies in its texture: a perfectly chewy interplay of butter-softened flour and baked oats. When it comes to cutting calories with our cookie consumption, we'd rather enjoy a first-rate cookie in a slightly smaller portion than eat an oversized and otherwise lackluster specimen. These are just like your mom used to make, only with an extra pinch of sea salt, which plays off the chocolaty sweetness in mysterious and magical ways. Serve with a jet-cold glass of milk (but you don't need us to tell you that).

You'll Need:

- 1 cup flour
- 1 cup rolled oats
- ¾ tsp baking powder
- ½ tsp baking soda
- ½ tsp salt
- ⅓ cup butter, softened
- 1 extra-large egg
- 1 tsp vanilla extract
- ½ cup light brown sugar
- ½ cup sugar
- ½ cup dark chocolate chips

How to Make It:

- Preheat the oven to 375°F.
- Combine the flour, oats, baking powder, baking soda, and salt in a large mixing bowl. In a separate mixing bowl, beat the butter, egg, vanilla, and both sugars until you have a uniform consistency. Add the flour mixture to the bowl, mixing gently to combine. Mix in the chocolate chips.
- Cover a cookie sheet with nonstick spray. Drop the dough on the sheet by generous tablespoons, keeping the cookies at least 2 inches apart. Bake for 10 to 12 minutes, just until the edges of the cookies begin to brown. Cool for a few minutes before eating.

Makes about 14 cookies.

Per Cookie
$0.20
200 calories
8 g fat
(4.5 g saturated)
18 g sugars

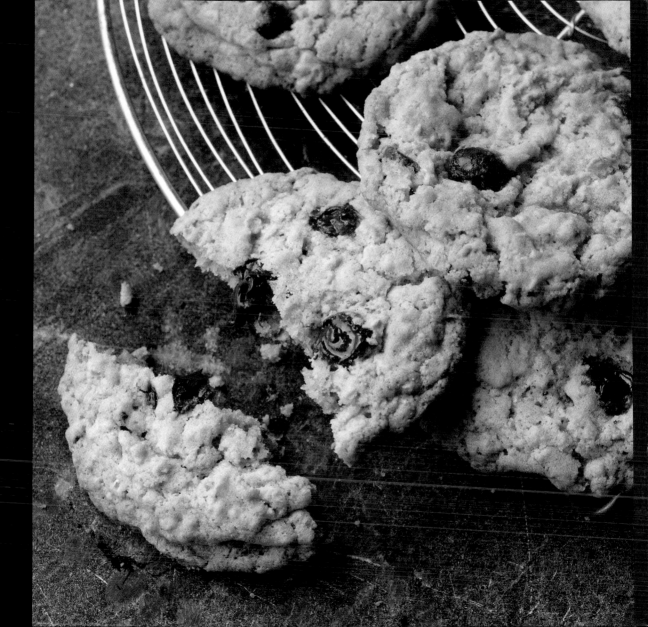

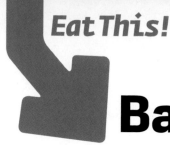

Banana Pudding

Allen & Son in Chapel Hill, North Carolina, may have achieved its renown by hickory-smoking pork shoulders into tender, juicy submission, but turns out this 'cue shack knows a thing or two about the sweet stuff, too. Its dessert menu reads like an encyclopedia entry on Southern comfort food: pecan pie, key lime pie, coconut-chess pie, peach cobbler. They save the best, though, for the last day of the work week: a sweet, custardy banana pudding that is the measuring stick by which all others should be judged. This is our tribute to that Friday-only phenom.

You'll Need:

- ½ cup plus 2 Tbsp sugar
- ⅓ cup all-purpose flour
- 2 cups 2% milk
- 3 eggs, separated
- 1 tsp vanilla extract

Pinch of salt

- 4 large ripe bananas, sliced
- ½ box (12 oz) vanilla wafers (about 35 wafers)

How to Make It:

- Preheat the oven to 375°F.

- Combine the ½ cup of sugar, the flour, milk, egg yolks, vanilla, and salt in a medium saucepan. Cook over low heat, whisking occasionally, for about 12 minutes, until the mixture thickens into a pudding.

- Place the egg whites in a mixing bowl and beat with an electric mixer until thick, stiff peaks have formed. Fold in the 2 table-spoons of sugar and mix for another few seconds to incorporate. (The meringue can also be whipped by hand with a whisk in a cold aluminum mixing bowl, but be prepared for a bit of a workout.)

- Layer the bottom of an 8" x 8" baking dish or oven-safe bowl with half of the bananas, then top with half the cookies. Repeat to form two layers of wafers and bananas, then pour the pudding over the top. Spread the meringue over the pudding. Bake for 10 to 12 minutes, until the meringue is golden brown.

Makes 8 servings

Per Serving

$0.65

290 calories
7 g fat
(2 g saturated)
36 g sugars

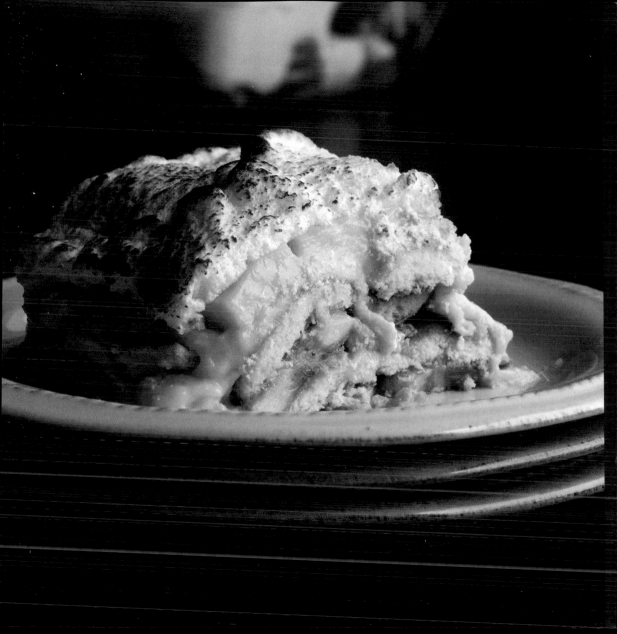

Ricotta Cheesecake with Warm Blueberries

The name says it all: a sugary, fat-laden slice of cake made almost entirely of cheese that we just can't get enough of. Go figure. This version is cut with ricotta for a light, creamy texture, and the warm blueberries lend a delicious dose of brain-boosting anthocyanins.

You'll Need:

- 8 oz graham crackers
- 6 Tbsp (¾ stick) butter, melted
- 1 container (12 oz) part-skim ricotta, drained
- 2 packages (8 oz each) light cream cheese, softened
- ¾ cup + 2 Tbsp sugar
- Grated zest and juice of 1 lemon
- 3 eggs
- 1 bag (16 oz) frozen blueberries

How to Make It:

- Preheat the oven to 350°F. Cover the outside of a 9" springform pan with a layer of aluminum foil.
- Grind the graham crackers in a food processor. Add the melted butter and whiz again. Pour the crumb mixture over the bottom (not the sides) of the pan and use a measuring cup to press them firmly into the pan. Bake for about 15 minutes, until the crust is a deep-brown shade.
- Blend the ricotta, cream cheese, ¾ cup of sugar, and lemon zest in the food processor until smooth. Add the eggs and pulse a few times.
- Pour the cheese mixture over the crust in the pan. Place the pan in a baking dish. Pour enough hot water into the dish to come halfway up the sides of the pan. Bake until the cheesecake is golden and the center of the cake moves slightly when the pan is gently shaken, about 1 hour.
- Cool for an hour on the counter, then refrigerate until the cheesecake is cold, at least 4 hours.
- While the cheesecake cools, combine the blueberries, lemon juice, and 2 tablespoons of sugar in a saucepan. Simmer for 5 minutes, until the blueberries begin to pop and become syrupy. Cut the cake into wedges and serve with a generous scoop of the blueberries over the top.

Makes 10 servings

Per Serving
$1.96
360 calories
19 g fat
(8 g saturated)
40 g carbs

SECRET WEAPON

Citrus Zest

The juice inside lemons, limes, and oranges isn't the fruits' only prized possession. The fragrant rind is home to the most intense citrus flavor of all and works great when stirred into everything from borscht to brownies. The best way to get it off is with a microplane, but the fine side of a cheese grater also works. Just be sure to stop as soon as you see the white pith emerge—its bitter notes can sink an otherwise tasty dish.

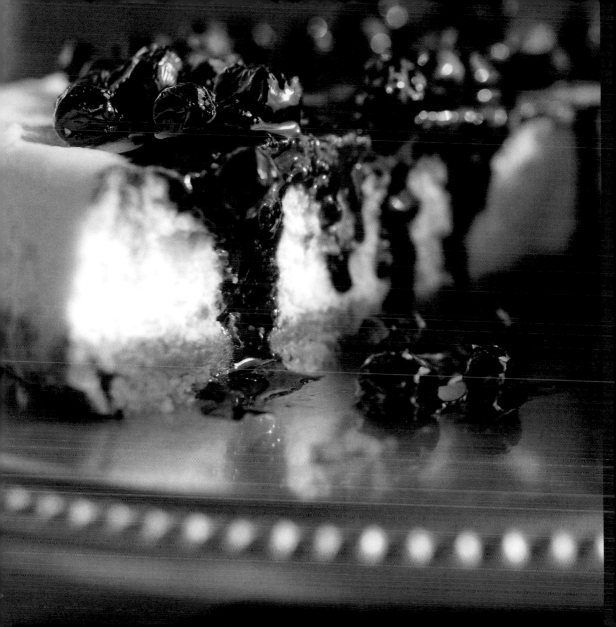

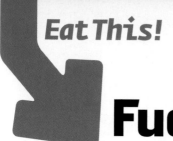

Eat This!

Fudgy Brownies

Low-calorie bakers have tried every trick in the book to come up with a "healthy" brownie: butter substitute, egg substitute, sugar substitute. One well-known cook even makes his brownies with mashed black beans. No thanks. Make a batch of brownies like that and you're likely to eat half a pan and still not feel satisfied. We'd rather get it right—with a restrained amount of butter and sugar and a dose of good dark chocolate— and offer a delicious square to devour than deal with the possibility of leaving you disappointed.

You'll Need:

- ½ cup (1 stick) butter
- 2 oz semisweet dark chocolate, chopped
- ¾ cup sugar
- ½ cup unsweetened cocoa powder
- 1½ tsp vanilla
- 3 eggs
- ½ cup all-purpose flour
- 1 tsp baking powder
- ¾ tsp salt
- ½ cup chopped walnuts (optional)

How to Make It:

- Preheat the oven to 350°F.
- Melt the butter and chocolate together in a pan set over low heat. Stir in the sugar, cocoa, and vanilla and remove from the heat. Add the eggs, flour, baking powder, and salt and whisk until smooth. Stir in the walnuts if using.
- Pour the batter into an 8" x 8" baking pan coated with a bit of nonstick spray. Spread the batter out into an even layer. Bake for 20 to 25 minutes, until a toothpick inserted in the center comes out nearly clean. (If you like your brownies less fudgy, bake a few extra minutes, until the toothpick comes out perfectly clean.)

Makes 12 brownies

Per Brownie
$0.46
200 calories
12.5 g fat
(6 g saturated)
16 g sugars

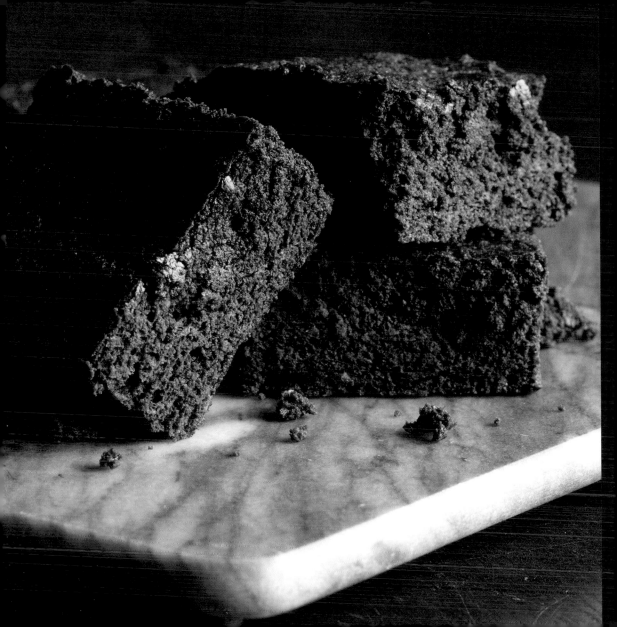

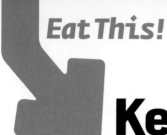

Key Lime Pie

This is the easiest pie in the history of baking. Mix, pour, bake, devour. Simple as that. If you can't find bottled Key lime juice (or fresh Key limes) in your local supermarket, you can have Amazon.com send you a 16-ounce bottle of Nellie & Joe's Key West Lime Juice for about $5. In a pinch, regular lime juice will do, even if the majority of south Floridians would cry foul.

You'll Need:

- 2 eggs
- 2 egg whites
- ½ cup Key lime juice
- 1½ tsp grated lime zest
- 1 can (14 oz) low-fat sweetened condensed milk
- 1 graham cracker crust (6 oz)
- 1½ cups low-fat whipped topping

How to Make It:

- Preheat the oven to 350°F. Beat the eggs and egg whites with a whisk or a mixer until blended. Stir in the juice, zest, and milk and beat until well blended.
- Pour the mixture into the crust. Bake on the center oven rack for about 20 minutes, until the center is set but still wobbly (it will firm up as it cools). Allow the pie to cool on the counter, then cover with plastic wrap and refrigerate for at least 2 hours. Before eating, spread the whipped topping evenly over the filling.

Makes 8 servings

Key limes have an intense tart flavor that standard limes just can't match. If you do use regular lime, add some extra zest to intensify the citrus kick.

LEFTOVER♥LOVE

Now that you've got all that extra Key lime juice, what to do with it? Try one of these with your new citrus supply:

- Mix equal parts curry powder, Key lime juice, and tomato paste. Slow cook chicken chunks and chickpeas in the sauce.
- Mix 2 tablespoons of juice with a half stick of softened butter. Top grilled fish and meat with it.
- Make a Key lime martini by shaking 1 part juice, 1 part simple syrup, and 2 parts vanilla vodka.

Per Serving
$1.34
330 calories
10 g fat
(5 g saturated)
39 g sugars

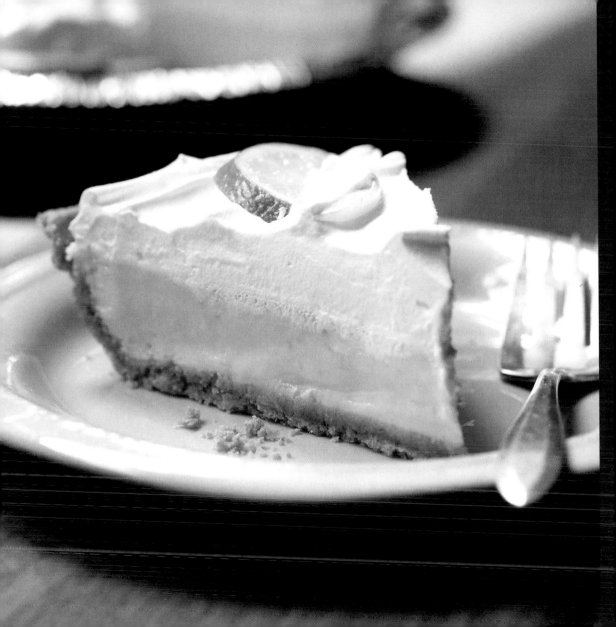

Eat This!

Grilled Fruit
Kebabs with Yogurt & Honey

The heat of the grill does something magical to fruit, teasing out natural sugars, softening flesh, and adding an element of smoke and char that transforms the average into something otherworldly. Tack on a cool yogurt sauce and you'll forget about the choco-bombs and sugar-fests that normally qualify as dessert; you'll also forget that you're eating one of the healthiest desserts on the planet.

You'll Need:

- 2 peaches, peeled, pitted, and chopped into ¾" pieces
- 2 cups pineapple chopped into ¾" pieces
- 2 cups watermelon chopped into ¾" pieces
- 4 metal skewers (or wooden skewers soaked in cold water for 20 minutes)
- ½ cup 2% Greek yogurt
- 2 Tbsp honey
- 2 Tbsp chopped fresh mint

How to Make It:

- Preheat a grill or grill pan over medium heat. Thread the fruit onto the skewers, alternating between peaches, pineapple, and watermelon so that each skewer has a colorful variety of fruit.
- Grill for about 8 minutes, turning occasionally, until the fruit is nicely caramelized.
- Combine the yogurt with the honey and drizzle over the skewers. Garnish with fresh mint.

Makes 4 servings

Mix up the fruit based on the season and what looks best in the market. Mangos, grapes, plums, apricots, and pretty much any firm-flesh fruits grill up beautifully.

Per Serving
$1.76
140 calories
1 g fat
(0 g saturated)
29 g sugars

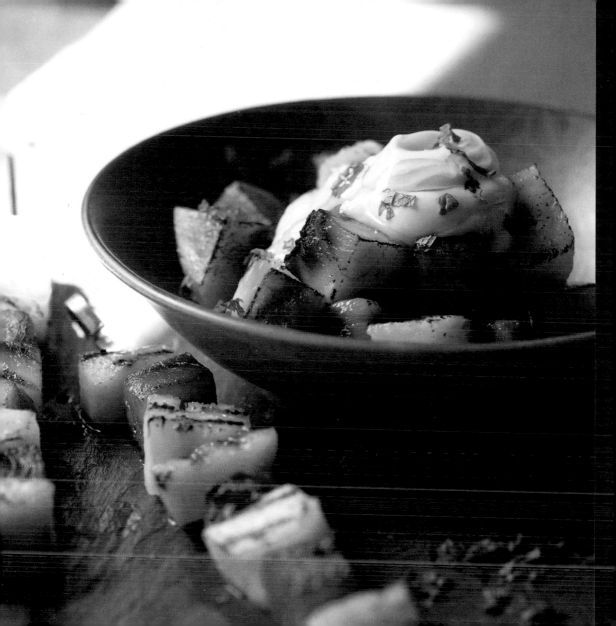

Tiramisu

Tiramisu is like guacamole and pizza: It's hard to have a truly bad version of it. The basic composition is so fundamentally delicious, even an ill-prepared rendition is still pretty damn satisfying. Unfortunately, that rule doesn't hold true for nutritional virtue, which tends to suffer in inverse proportion to the deliciousness of a given tiramisu. This version bucks that trend, ditching the high-cal constituents—egg yolks and mascarpone—in favor of a lighter treatment of beaten egg whites and whipped cream cheese, an approach that yields an ethereal, but still rich and satisfying dessert.

You'll Need:

- 3 egg whites
- ¼ cup confectioners' sugar
- ½ cup whipped cream cheese, softened at room temperature
- ½ cup strong espresso (or 1 cup strong coffee)
- ½ cup coffee liqueur such as Kahlua or Tia Maria
- ½ package (7 oz) ladyfingers or 4 cups cubed angel food cake
- 1 oz dark chocolate, finely shaved
- Espresso grounds or cocoa powder (optional)

How to Make It:

- Beat the egg whites until they form soft peaks. Add the sugar and lightly beat it into the whites. Place the cream cheese in a large bowl and fold in half of the whipped whites. Once fully incorporated, lightly fold in the remaining whites.

- Combine the espresso and coffee liqueur. Place a layer of ladyfingers (or angel food cake, if using) in the bottom of 4 wine or martini glasses. Spoon enough of the coffee mixture over them to soak the ladyfingers thoroughly. Divide the cream cheese mixture among the glasses, then top each with a good pile of dark chocolate shavings. Garnish with a dusting of espresso grounds if you like.

Makes 4 servings

Ladyfingers—short, stubby sponge cakes— are traditional here, but angel food cake provides a similarly soft, absorbent base and keeps the calorie count a touch lower.

Per Serving
$2.02
260 calories
6 g fat
(4 g saturated)
23 g sugars

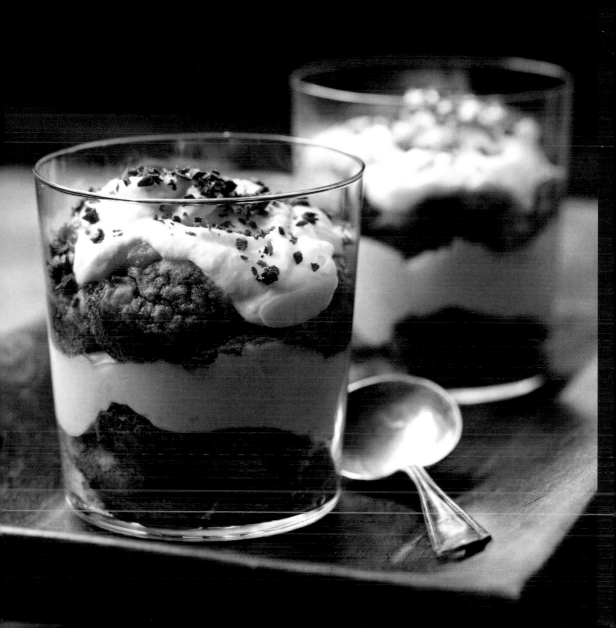

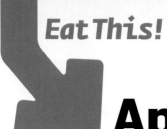
Apple Pie with Crunch Topping

Most apple pies are made with two crusts, one as the base, the other as the top, doubling up on the impact of the refined carbs and cheap fats that make up the pastry. Here, we replace the second crust with a crunchy topping made of oats, chopped almonds, and brown sugar, providing a perfect textural counterpoint to the soft baked apples while actually bolstering the overall nutrition of the dessert.

You'll Need:

- 2 Granny Smith apples, peeled, cored, and sliced
- 2 Gala apples, peeled, cored, and sliced
- ⅓ cup granulated sugar
- ½ cup unsweetened applesauce
- 1 Tbsp flour
- Juice of 1 lemon
- 1½ tsp cinnamon
- 1 frozen pie shell, thawed
- ¼ cup chopped almonds
- ¼ cup light brown sugar
- ¼ cup rolled oats
- 2 Tbsp cold butter, diced

How to Make It:

- Preheat the oven to 375°F.
- Combine the apples, granulated sugar, applesauce, flour, lemon juice, and 1 teaspoon of the cinnamon in a large mixing bowl. Stir to thoroughly combine, then scrape into the pie shell. (Depending on the size of your apples, this may make more filling than you need. The apples should rise slightly over the pie shell, mounding in the center.)
- Combine the almonds, brown sugar, oats, butter, and remaining ½ teaspoon cinnamon in a bowl. Use your fingers to help break up the butter and mix with the other ingredients.
- Sprinkle the topping evenly over the pie. Place on the middle rack and bake for 45 to 50 minutes, until the apples are soft and the crust is golden brown. Cool before slicing and serving with scoops of vanilla ice cream.

Makes 6 servings

Per Serving
$1.41
360 calories
14 g fat
(5 g saturated)
38 g sugars

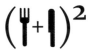

MEAL MULTIPLIER

Most people prefer their apple pie with a little something on top. Here are three great low-calorie ways to gild the lily.

- A 130-calorie scoop of Breyers Vanilla
- For a leaner add-on, try a bit of 2% Greek yogurt spiked with honey
- For a more elegant counterpoint to the sweetness of the apples, a spoonful of crème fraîche (French-style sour cream) makes a lovely topping for this pie

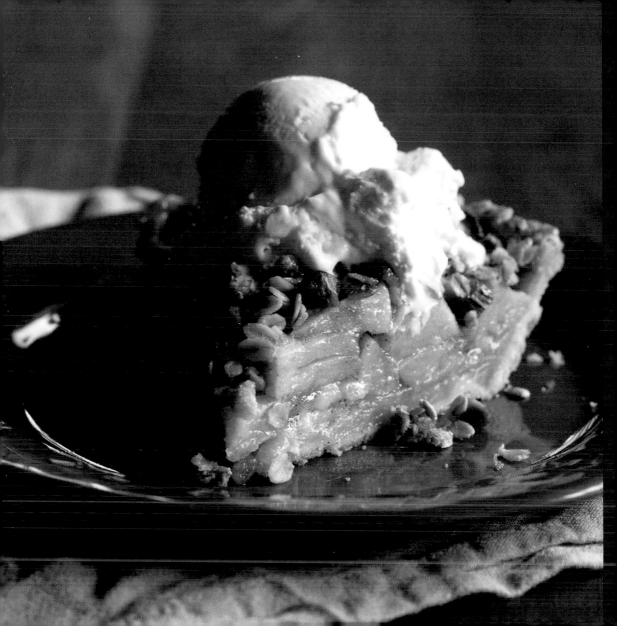

Molten Chocolate Cake

The idea of baking and frosting a multitiered chocolate cake is daunting for most, but these little self-contained parcels of joy are the lazy man's cake, the type of dessert that makes a non-baker feel like a pastry king when they emerge from the oven, pregnant with a tide of melted chocolate. Crack the middle and watch the flood of lava flow freely onto your plate—and eventually into your eagerly awaiting mouth. Did we mention these have only 360 calories?

You'll Need:

- 4 oz bittersweet chocolate (at least 60 percent cacao), plus 4 chunks for the cake centers
- 2 Tbsp butter
- 2 eggs
- 2 egg yolks
- ¼ cup sugar
- Pinch of salt
- 2 Tbsp flour
- 1 tsp vanilla extract
- ½ Tbsp instant coffee or espresso (optional)

How to Make It:

- Preheat the oven to 425°F. Lightly butter four 6-ounce ramekins or custard cups.
- Bring a few cups of water to a boil in a medium saucepan over low heat. Place a glass mixing bowl over the pan (but not touching the water) and add the chocolate and butter. Cook, stirring occasionally, until both the chocolate and butter have fully melted. Keep warm.
- Use an electric mixer to beat the eggs, egg yolks, sugar, and salt until pale yellow and thick, about 5 minutes. Stir in the melted chocolate mixture, the flour, vanilla, and instant coffee if using.
- Pour the mixture into the prepared ramekins. Stick one good chunk of chocolate in the center of each ramekin. Bake the cakes on the center rack for 8 to 10 minutes, until the exterior is just set (the center should still be mostly liquid). The cakes can be eaten straight from the ramekins, but it's more dramatic to slide them onto plates (after letting them rest for a minute or two), where the molten chocolate can flow freely.

Makes 4 servings

Per Serving
$1.20
320 calories
22 g fat
(11 g saturated)
31 g carbs

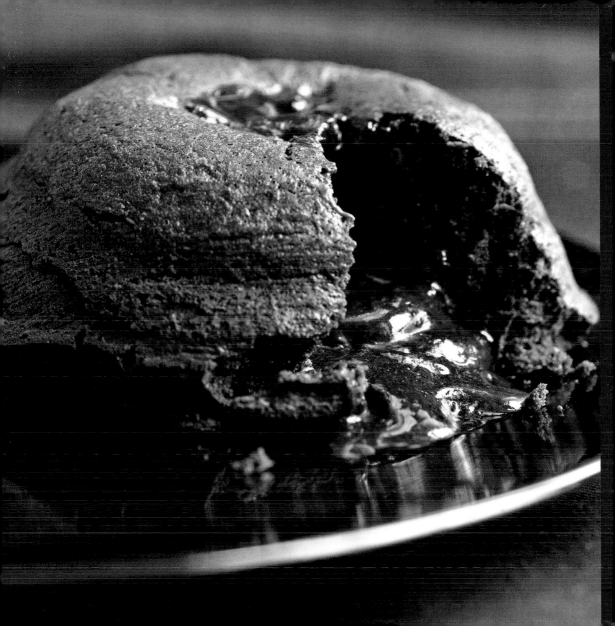

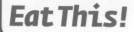

Blueberry-Peach Cobbler

By the time the dog days of summer arrive, you're no longer dreaming of warm brownies or chocolate cake; you want something that both refreshes and celebrates the season, and this cobbler does both. At its core are the two greatest summer fruits of all time (which also happen to be two of the healthiest ingredients on the planet, bursting with fiber and potent antioxidants), baked into a state of sweet intensity and topped with crisp-tender biscuits, perfect for soaking up all those lovely fruit juices.

You'll Need:

- 2 lbs peaches, peeled, pitted, and each cut into 6 wedges
- 1 cup blueberries
- ¼ cup + 2 Tbsp sugar
- 2 tsp cornstarch
- Juice of ½ lemon
- Salt
- 1 cup all-purpose flour
- 4 Tbsp cold butter, cut into cubes
- ¾ tsp baking powder
- ¼ tsp baking soda
- ⅓ cup plain 2% Greek yogurt
- 1 Tbsp brown sugar

How to Make It:

- Preheat the oven to 350°F. Combine the peaches, blueberries, the ¼ cup sugar, the cornstarch, lemon juice, and a pinch of salt in an 8" x 8" baking dish. Mix thoroughly with a large spoon.

- Combine the 2 tablespoons sugar, the flour, butter, baking powder, baking soda, and ¼ teaspoon of salt in a mixing bowl. Use your fingers to break up the butter and mash with the flour until the consistency is like coarse meal. Add the yogurt and stir gently to create a shaggy dough (don't overmix or you will have tough biscuits).

- Divide the dough into 6 equal mounds. Arrange the mounds out over the peaches and sprinkle with the brown sugar.

- Bake for about 20 minutes, until the peaches are bubbling and the biscuits are golden brown.

Makes 6 servings

Per Serving
$1.36
310 calories
9 g fat
(5 g saturated)
32 g sugars

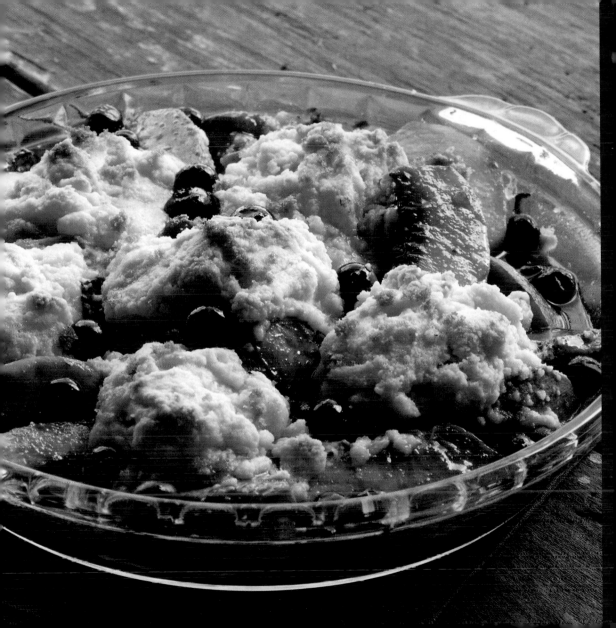

Grilled
Banana Split

There truly is something transformative about the way the banana emerges from a grill grate. The warm caramelized fruit adds a layer of sexiness to the classic split, especially in the way the heat of the banana plays off the chill of the ice cream. Salted peanuts add crunch and contrast while chocolate doubles down on the decadence. And yet all of this can be yours for the low, low price of just 320 calories!

You'll Need:

- 2 bananas, unpeeled
- 2 Tbsp light brown sugar
- 4 scoops vanilla ice cream
- 4 Tbsp chocolate sauce, heated
- 4 Tbsp roasted and salted peanuts, roughly chopped

How to Make It:

- Preheat a grill or grill pan over medium-high heat. Cut the bananas in half lengthwise, being sure to leave each half in the peel. Coat the cut sides of the bananas with the brown sugar, using your fingers to press the sugar into the flesh of the fruit. Place the bananas on the grill, cut sides down, and grill for about 3 minutes, until the sugar caramelizes and forms a deep-brown crust. Flip and grill for another 2 to 3 minutes, until the bananas are warmed all the way through but not mushy.
- Remove the peels from the bananas and place each half in the bottom of a bowl. Top with a scoop of ice cream, a good drizzle of hot chocolate sauce, and a handful of peanuts.

Makes 4 servings

For the best possible splits, the bananas should be ripe, but not soft.

Per Serving
$0.96
320 calories
12 g fat
(5 g saturated)
38 g sugars

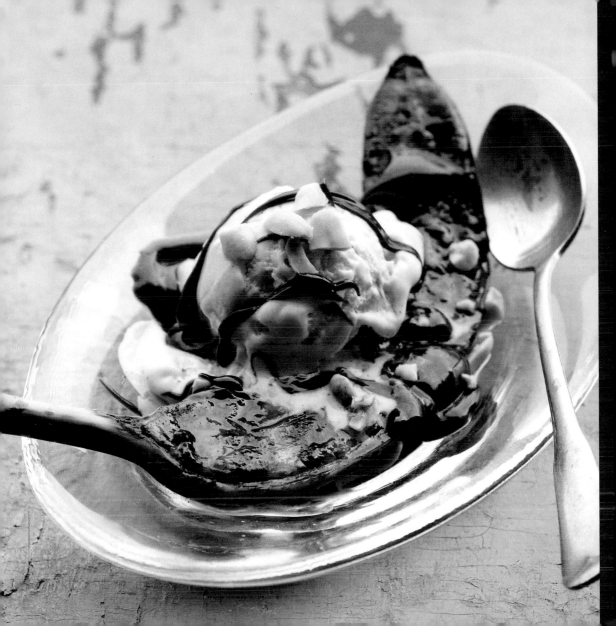

Index